RUNNING
MADE

Lisa Jackson & Susie Whalley

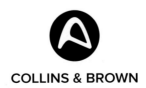

COLLINS & BROWN

WHAT READERS HAVE TO SAY ABOUT
RUNNING MADE EASY

Running Made Easy

This edition published in 2014
by Collins and Brown
10 Southcombe Street
London W14 0RA

An imprint of Anova Books
First published in Great Britain in 2004

Distributed in the United States and Canada by
Sterling Publishing Co, 387 Park Avenue South,
New York, 10016-8810, USA

The publishers have made every reasonable
effort to contact all copyright holders. Any
errors that may have occurred are inadvertent
and anyone who for any reason has not been
contacted is invited to write to the publishers so
that a full acknowledgement may be made in
subsequent editions of this work.

A CIP catalogue for this book is available from
the British Library.

ISBN 978-1-90939-777-4

Picture credits:
Photograph of Lisa by Graham Williams
Photographs courtesy of Shutterstock /Giovanni
G p11, / Warren Goldswain front cover, p19,
p.89, / Maridav p31, / dotshock p41, / Dirima
p51, / MJTH p67, / Gabi Moisa p141, /
wavebreakmedia p169, / Ammentorp
Photography p175, / Dirima p203, / Odua
Images p207.
Photo on page 193 and 199 courtesy of
Action Photo.
Photos on pages 21-2, 24-5 and 27 courtesy of
Slimming World.
Illustrator Drew Gilbert

10 9 8 7 6 5 4 3 2 1

Reproduction by Mission Productions Ltd,
Hong Kong
Printed and bound by Times, Malaysia

LISA JACKSON is a clinical hypnotherapist
and Contributing Editor to UK-based *Women's
Running* magazine. An extremely reluctant
convert to running, she's now an ardent
evangelist and has walked/run over 50
marathons and ultramarathons in fancy dress.
Lisa is currently writing her second running
book, *It's Not About The Time You Do, It's About
The Time You Have*. Born in South Africa, she
lives in London with her husband Graham.

LISA'S THANKS
This book is dedicated to my beloved mother,
Leone Jackson, who was tragically killed, aged
68, while training to run the Medoc Marathon
with our family, and my Aunt Rosie, my trusty
companion during eight marathons, who sadly
died of lung cancer in 2011. Both of them
encouraged my entire family to run and they
continue to inspire us. I'd also like to thank my
husband Graham Williams (who's done over
20 marathons and ultramarathons with me –
entirely against his will), Loren Jackson, Anthony
Jackson, Bridget and Kent Robinson, Ian Beach,
Ivy Shakespeare and Sarah Owen. And finally,
thanks to the dozens of you who shared your
amazing stories with us.

SUSIE WHALLEY is a writer, runner and
mum to two boys. Having discovered running in
her mid-20s after a long lapse, she has now run
five London Marathons and one New York City
Marathon, along with numerous shorter races.
She lives in London with her husband Adam
and sons Stanley and Alf.

SUSIE'S THANKS
Thanks to my dad for inspiring me to start
running and encouraging me all the way.
He's a great runner (3:20, Robin Hood
Marathon, Nottingham, 1985) and a great role
model – I only hope I'm as fit as him when I'm
73! Thanks also to my husband Adam, the
ultimate unwilling runner, who took a leap of
faith by running his (one and only!) marathon
with me, and who supported me through
writing this book. Thanks also to all of you
fabulous readers who've contacted us. To
know we've helped you out makes it all feel
so worthwhile.

The exercise programmes in this book are
intended for people in good health – if you
have a medical condition or are pregnant,
or have any other health concerns, consult
your GP before starting out.

CONTENTS

GET TO KNOW US

We've written our book *Running Made Easy* because we're bursting to tell you about the joys of running and the in-love-with-life way it can make you feel. Turn the page to find out how we got hooked – and how we can help you do the same ...

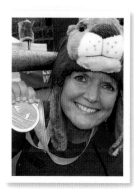

LISA JACKSON, JOURNALIST AND CLINICAL HYPNOTHERAPIST

Running pace

Think of the slowest runner you know – then think twice as slow!

Running CV

I'm a late-onset runner. For 30 years I simply detested exercise. Then, in June 1998, I was blown away by the electrifying atmosphere of a 5K (3 mile) race that I'd been cajoled into doing. Soon afterwards, I entered the Great North Run, at that time the world's biggest half-marathon, and again was bowled over by the thrill of having dared to run that far. Six months later, I completed the London Marathon and from then on, I was well and truly hooked.

I've since run 48 other marathons and two 56-mile/90K ultramarathons in dream destinations such as Jerusalem, Hong Kong, Stockholm, New York, Paris and Athens. My ultimate goal? Joining the 100 Marathon Club.

What I wish I'd known about running before I started

I wish I'd known about the ecstasy of running – the feeling of flushed wellbeing I get after a training run I begged myself not to have to do, but did anyway; the incomparable feeling of crossing the finish line in a race, having used up every last ounce of willpower to get there. I wish I'd known about the friends I'd make. If I'd known these things, I'd most definitely have started running at 20 – not 30!

How writing Running Made Easy has changed my life

Before writing this book, I had no idea how many people out there felt just as intimidated as I did about taking up running, believing, erroneously, that it simply wasn't suitable for tortoise types like us. So when emails flooded in from readers who said our book had given them bagloads of confidence and generally made them fall in love with life again, I was deeply moved. This has inspired me to gain a coaching qualification from British Athletics and train as a clinical hypnotherapist, which has meant I've been privileged to be able to continue to help others change their lives for good. I have also spent the past three years running and writing about marathons in the UK and abroad in my capacity as 'the world's slowest marathon correspondent' for Women's Running magazine. Having come last in no fewer than three marathons, I'm uniquely placed to encourage other runners to ditch their need for speed, don a fancy-dress outfit and run a marathon – just for the heck of it!

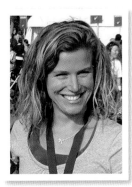

SUSIE WHALLEY, JOURNALIST

Running pace
Once fairly sprightly and competitive –
now, with two children and less youthful
energy, it's a bit more 'middle aged'!

Running CV
My earliest memories of running are of
trotting off down country lanes with my
dad to fetch the morning baguette on
family holidays in France. Even aged
eight, with little legs that could barely
keep up, I was desperate to become
a runner like him. At school I loved
sports days, and every April I'd watch
the London Marathon with tears in my
eyes, dreaming of taking part.

My ambitions were shelved at
university (too much time at the bar!),
so when I decided to start training for
the marathon aged 25, it felt pretty
tough. But I did it, loved it, and amazingly
it's now 15 years down the line and I've
run a total of six marathons and heaps
of other races since. Being a runner has
become a really big part of who I am
and I wouldn't change that for the world.

Proudest moment
Rounding the corner to run up The
Mall towards the finish line of my first
London Marathon, holding hands with
my great friend Louise. With the crowd
cheering us on, and the finish line in
sight, knowing we were going to make
it was just the most fantastic feeling in
the world. Another is crossing the finish
line of the Windsor Half Marathon,
hand in hand with my lovely sons.
It's the longest distance I've run since
becoming a mum, and Stanley and
Alf were proud to join me on the home
straight and run the last 50m together.

Most embarrassing moment
Hmmm, quite a few. Sprinting for the
finish line in a race only to be told I'd
gone the wrong way and having to
retrace my steps. Trying to discreetly
breastfeed my son soon after finishing
a 10K race while wearing a sports bra.
I could go on ...

What running has taught me
To love, respect and listen to my body
and to be grateful for all the hundreds
of miles my legs have carried me. I've
also learnt that running can be a
lifelong passion that gives you just
what you need, just when you need it –
regardless of how much your life and
your ambitions change. Now in my 40s,
I use running to maintain a bit of
identity amid the happy chaos of
family life, and to encourage my boys
to get active, too. But regardless of all
that's changed, what remains the
same is the amazing way running still
makes me feel – alive, energized and
ready to enjoy the day ahead.

WONDERING IF RUNNING IS REALLY FOR YOU, OR WHY YOU'RE MORE LIKELY TO STICK TO OUR PROGRAMME THAN ANY OTHER YOU'VE ALREADY TRIED? WE'RE HERE TO ANSWER ALL YOUR QUESTIONS, BANISH ALL YOUR DOUBTS, AND SET YOU ON THE ROAD TO RUNAWAY SUCCESS ...

1. GET READY

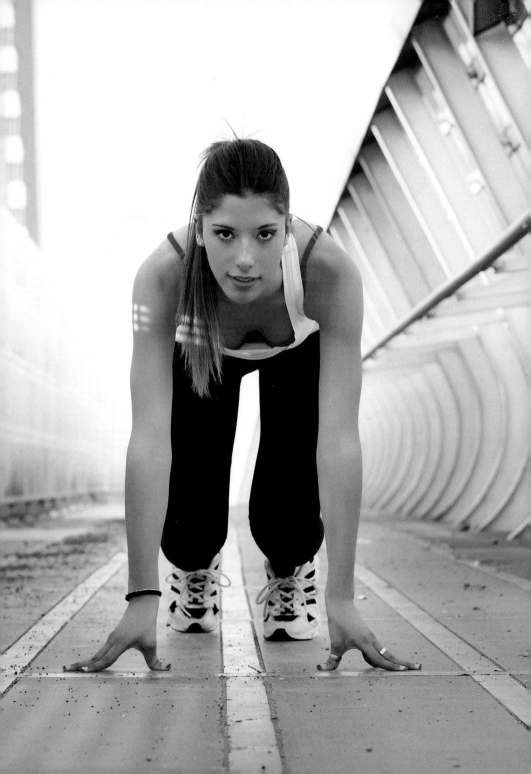

CAN YOU SPARE A MINUTE?

Yes, we do mean just 60 seconds. If so, you've got what it takes to do something that has the power to shape up your whole life and totally transform you, from your quads to your brain cells and beyond. This is an activity that will make you feel passionate, alive, energized, joyful and confident in a way that no jumbo croissant or retail therapy ever could. It can turn you into a hero for a day, and get thousands of people chanting your name. And it's something that you've known how to do since childhood, but have probably neglected to do since you grew up. Something that's blindingly obvious, easy to fit into your day – and free. Quite simply, it's running.

BUT WILL IT WORK FOR ME?

Of course, if you give it a chance. The best thing about running is that it can give you whatever you need – whether that's a better body, quiet time to think, or something more radical like the confidence to make life-changing decisions or tackle an 'I didn't think I had it in me' challenge. But in order for running to work for you, you need to approach it in the right way. Try to run too far, too fast (as you may have done in the past) and you'll find

yourself doubled over with exhaustion, giving up before you even get to the good bits. But do it right and it's actually amazingly easy – providing you know where to start. And that's where *Running Made Easy* comes in. We've developed something called 'The 60-Second-Secret Plan', which we believe is the very best way to ease you painlessly into running. If you've barely run a step in your life – or even if you've been running half-heartedly for years – The 60-Second-Secret Plan will take you back to basics and help you build a solid fitness foundation that will enable you to achieve all your goals. Follow this plan and you'll fall in love with running – for life. Guaranteed! It's all about starting small but aiming big. About learning to combine walking with 60-second bursts of running (as fast or slow as you like) and building up from there. It'll take you wherever you want to go – from minute to mile to marathon.

WHY RUN?
▶▶▶▶▶▶▶▶▶▶▶▶▶▶▶▶▶▶▶▶▶▶▶▶

Apart from helping you look and feel fantastic, running can massively improve your health, something most of us in the Western world really need to do. A worrying 80% of adults in England don't get enough exercise, and we're suffering from a host of health problems related to this lack of physical activity. The good news is that running can help stop many of them in their tracks. Here's the evidence to prove it:

161,000 deaths a year in the UK are caused by cardiovascular disease (mainly heart disease and stroke). That's around four out of every ten deaths. (*British Heart Foundation*)

50% is how much you can reduce your risk of heart disease if you're physically active. (*British Heart Foundation*)

63% is how much you can reduce your risk of stroke if you run regularly for 20–40 minutes, three to five times a week. (*Medicine and Science In Sports and Exercise Journal*)

1.4 billion adults worldwide are overweight and at least 400 million are obese. (*World Health Organization*)

100% is how sure we are that you'll lose weight if you exercise regularly and reduce your calorie intake.

31% is how much higher your risk of developing breast cancer is, if you are a woman who is post-menopausal and obese. (*European Prospective Investigation of Cancer*)

30% is how much you can reduce your risk of breast cancer if you exercise on a regular basis. (*University of Bristol research*)

12,000 people a year in the UK might avoid getting cancer if they maintained a healthy body weight. (*International Journal of Cancer*)

382 million people worldwide have diabetes, with up to 95% of them suffering from type-2 diabetes, which is often associated with being overweight. (*International Diabetes Federation*)

Up to 80% of type-2 diabetes is preventable by adopting a healthy diet and increasing physical activity. (*International Diabetes Federation*)

58% is how much participants in a study reduced their risk of getting type-2 diabetes by, by exercising, on average, for 30 minutes per day. (*Joslin Diabetes Center*)

30–40 minutes of weight-bearing exercise (such as running) three to four times a week can help to prevent osteoporosis. (*Osteoporosis Australia*)

WHY GO BACK TO BASICS?

Because we know there's nothing more frustrating than programmes that ask too much of you, such as those that expect you to be able to run for 10 minutes on day one when you know you just can't. Because we know that the last time you ran for the bus, you probably missed it. Because we know runners who were so terrified of exercising in public that they'd run only under the cover of darkness, or jog with a shopping bag so they could pretend they weren't running at all but merely in a rush to get to the supermarket! With this plan, it doesn't matter where you are now or how embarrassed and unfit you feel – you'll definitely be able to manage it. We promise.

SO WHY LISTEN TO US?

As fitness journalists, we have access to all the latest running research and the best experts, so we can give you the lowdown on the technical stuff. But that's not all this book is about. The fact is that we're runners ourselves, and we've learned things you can discover only by getting out there and running. Which means that whatever you're going through, we've been there, too.

And because one of us is a tortoise, a slow but sure runner who always gets to the end eventually, and the other a hare who loves tearing after the front runners, we know all about the challenges different types of running bring. Between us, we've made just about every mistake in the book. We know what it's like to shoot out of the door on the first day of your new fitness regime, so overenthusiastic that you attempt to run full-tilt for 20 minutes, only to wilt so badly after ten that you have to catch a taxi home. What it's like to go running in winter in a T-shirt and almost turn blue from the cold.

We know what it is like to be so late for a race that you hear the start gun go off while you're still stuck trying to pin on your race number. Or to break the biggest rule of all, and run a marathon in brand new trainers that turn your feet into a bubble wrap of blisters after the first mile.

We've also experienced pretty much every positive emotion running can arouse – the joy of achieving what you set out to do, the deep satisfaction of realizing you've been running three times a week for six months and it no longer feels like a struggle, and the pride in finishing a tough race you never thought you could.

Best of all, we're still running and loving every step. We try never to lose sight of the fact that running is fun, and that's why we do it. We know that as well as exercising our glutes, hamstrings and quads, each run should never fail to exercise 53 really important muscles that aren't used nearly often enough – the ones that make you smile!

> ## 'We try never to lose sight of the fact that running is fun, and that's why we do it'

NINE MIGHTY REASONS TO RUN

▶▶▶

1. Because you can indulge in chocolate (and other treats) without putting on weight.

2. Because it will give you so much confidence your friends will be wondering what has made the difference.

3. Because it will give you the energy to bound through your day and still have enough left over to last well into the night.

4. Because it will help banish cellulite, which means shorts will not just be for running.

5. Because the ear-to-ear grin that running gives you will make you totally irresistible.

6. Because being successful at running makes you realize you can dare to go after your dreams – however wild they may seem.

7. Because it'll make you feel young and help you turn back the clock without any artificial help.

8. Because you'll save money by not spending on 'miracle' diet books, expensive low-calorie foods and cigarettes.

9. Because it's so easy to fit into your life, it'll leave you plenty of time for all those other things you love to do.

WHAT EXACTLY WILL I LEARN?

Basically, how to run. And although it sounds simple, it does need to be learned. Which is where *Running Made Easy* comes in. We want to be with you every step of the way, and that's why this book is packed with all you need to know to help you achieve just about any running goal you might set yourself. We also want it to be really useful, which is why it's also a workbook that we hope you'll fill in regularly to help you track your progress and record your personal achievements, from the joy of going farther than you've ever gone before to the satisfaction of fitting into a smaller pair of jeans.

BUT WILL IT INSPIRE ME?

Yes, because you'll find this book is full of tips and advice from ordinary people just like you – and a few extraordinary ones, too, like the woman who lost half her bodyweight through running and the blind man who still dares to run. You'll learn what motivates people to run, what helps them stick at it when the going gets tough, and hear more about how they came to realize that, by running, they really could change their life for the better. It really is stirring stuff – we were amazed and we think you'll be, too.

This is also a book that devotes as much time to examining the mental and emotional benefits of running as the physical ones. It'll show you how you can use running as a self-help tool to calm yourself after a frantic day in the office, develop the self-esteem you'll never find at the bottom of a wine glass, and gain the body confidence that a new designer wardrobe can't deliver.

SO WHEN DO I START?

In a minute! Just one last thing. Always remember that whoever you are, and whatever your starting point, you can be a good runner – it's not about being fast or first, it's about achieving what you set out to do, whether that's one lap of the park, 10 minutes on the treadmill, or finishing your first race or marathon. But most of all, it's about having fun!

OUR PROMISE TO YOU

Running will make you:

- Happier

- Slimmer

- More successful

- More confident

- More assertive

- Sexier

- More positive

- Less stressed

Guaranteed!

'WHAT I WISH I'D KNOWN BEFORE I STARTED...'

NOT EVERYONE GETS TO READ A COPY OF *RUNNING MADE EASY* BEFORE EMBARKING ON THEIR FIRST RUN! HERE, A FEW RUNNERS SHARE THE MISTAKES THEY MADE, TO HELP STOP YOU FROM MAKING THEM, TOO.

I wish that someone had told me that at the start of every run, I'd have to be patient and wait for my body to warm up. I always set off feeling terrible, and my body would feel like it was shocked because one minute I'd been sitting on the sofa, and the next I was out running. But, if I stuck with it and gave myself time to get into my stride, it started to get a lot easier.'
Jill Hopper, 38, journalist, London

'It's good to plan a running route so you have some idea of where you're going. The first time I ran, I got lost and had to ask people the way home! I got on much better when I found some local running routes on the Internet. It also meant I knew exactly how far I was running which helped to motivate me.'
Will Fuller, 35, HR Manager, Surrey

'It took me a while to realize how much easier I'd find it running with someone. I'd get bored and lonely running by myself (music was the only thing that kept me going) but when I was with a friend, I could chat away quite happily which passed the time and meant I didn't really focus on the fact that I was finding it hard work.'
Lindsay Cunningham, 34, teacher, Hampshire

'Running gives you energy when you're tired, and helps you to eat more healthily. As a student nurse, I can be on my feet for 12 hours a day and I used to sometimes think I was too tired to go for a run, so would pick myself up by eating crisps and chocolate instead. But now I've realized that running is a brilliant way to de-stress, and when I've finished a run, I want to eat healthily rather than undo all my good work with junk food.'
Rose Danaher, 27, student nurse, London

'It would have been good to get my underwear sorted earlier on! When I took up running to train for a marathon, I did a few races wearing uncomfortable knickers, and ended up with really sore, chafed legs where the seams had rubbed. I eventually realized the fewer seams the better, and at times I even found it was best to go commando under my shorts!'
Rachel Roberts, 29, teacher, Cornwall

PREPARE TO SEE SOME TRULY STUNNING TRANSFORMATIONS. EACH OF THE TEN PEOPLE OVERLEAF HAS TAKEN A LEAP OF FAITH AND RUN THEIR WAY FROM FAT TO FIT – GAINING HEAPS OF CONFIDENCE ALONG THE WAY. BETWEEN THEM, THEY'VE LOST AN AMAZING 306KG (49ST 1½LB) – AND IF THEY CAN DO IT, YOU CAN, TOO!

2. GET INSPIRED

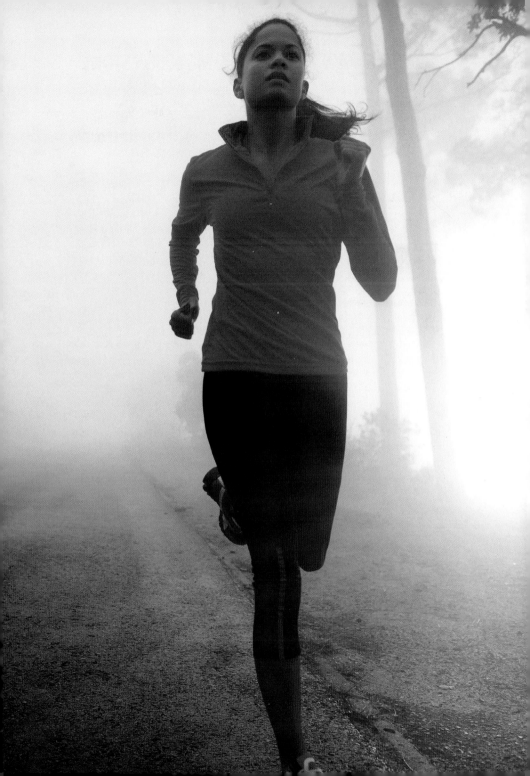

'RUNNING MADE EASY HELPED ME LOSE 5 STONE'

Dee Grimes, 31
After-school centre manager
Height 1.73m (5ft 8in)

Before	After
102kg (16st)	70kg (11st)
Dress size 18	Dress size 10/12

WEIGHT LOST 32KG (5ST)

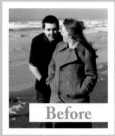
Before

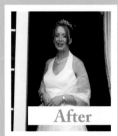
After

Thanks to *Running Made Easy*, I am a changed woman. It helped me go from being overweight and unfit to doing my first marathon in just 18 months. I had a weight problem all my life and as a child was painfully shy. It was a vicious circle. I knew I needed to exercise and slim down but I was too self-conscious to wear workout gear, so I remained overweight. It wasn't food that was the problem – I ate a healthy, vegetarian diet – just the lack of activity.

After I had my first child, Sean, my weight hit an all-time high of 102kg (16st). I felt awful. I hated buying clothes and going out. Three years later, I developed a blood clot in my lung, which made me realise I needed to change my lifestyle. I began to go out for walks and do pilates and gradually slimmed down to 89kg (14st).

That's when I bought a copy of *Running Made Easy*. It became my bible and I took it everywhere. I liked it so much I read it twice! I embarked on The 60-Second-Secret Plan. Soon afterwards, I signed up for the 10K (6-mile) Women's Mini-Marathon in Dublin. I had a great race and this spurred me on to keep running. And as I did so, the weight just kept falling off. By the time I got married, I was 70kg (11st).

Over the next year I completed six more races and finished the Dublin Marathon (42.2K/26.2 miles) in 4 hours. I've since had another child and running has helped me regain my pre-pregnancy figure. Before I read *Running Made Easy*, I thought running was only for athletes, but it helped me see that even if you're not super-fast and don't train every day you can still be proud to call yourself a runner.

HOW DEE DID IT
Training tip: 'Don't skip your rest days – your body needs them in order to recover from training sessions.'
Motivation tip: 'My motto is "Get up and out!" Don't give yourself time to think before starting an early morning training session – just head for the door and tell yourself you'll do just a few minutes. Once you get going you'll find you're happy to run for much longer than that.'

'THE RUNNING BUG TOOK HOLD OF ME'

Gill Hindmarsh, 55
Self-employed soft furnisher
Height 1.63m (5ft 4in)

Before	After
130kg (20st 7lb)	75kg (11st 12lb)

WEIGHT LOST 55KG (8ST 9LB)

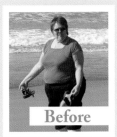

Before

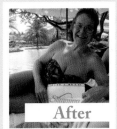

After

When I first decided I wanted to lose weight I was so determined that I joined my nearest Slimming World group as soon as I could. I initially felt embarrassed by my size but I received such a lovely, warm welcome and was made to feel like all my weight-loss dreams were achievable.

With the help of weekly group sessions and support from my consultant, I gradually lost 55kg (8st 9lb). I started to feel amazing and wanted to get active, so started off by going for walks. This progressed to speed walking and then occasionally some jogging. I entered the 5K (3 mile) Race for Life and ran it wearing a pink tutu and fairy wings, and my picture even made the local paper. The running bug took hold of me and soon I couldn't get enough. Although I was exercising more I never felt hungry and my consultant even told me to up my protein intake. I found this really helped with my running.

Losing the weight meant that I could walk and run much further without getting aches in my lower back – something that I used to really struggle with before. Now I don't get out of breath and can bend and reach easily. I can go up and down stairs as many times as I like. In fact, when I iron I take up each hanging item separately, just to keep moving!

The biggest joy in my whole life is to go for a run with my sons. It makes me feel so proud of myself because I know they are proud of me. I have so much energy now, some days I run, garden, cook, clean and tidy the house and I'm still on the go at 6pm. I feel half my age. Now I am fit and happy and I would like to progress my running even further. I have managed just over 10K (6 miles), so I am aiming for 15K and maybe even a half-marathon.

HOW GILL DID IT

Training tip: 'Having a good pair of leggings and the right layers for exercising really makes a difference. Being comfortable on a run is vital.'
Motivation tip: 'Take every run as it comes. Progressing little by little is a guaranteed way of seeing great results long term.'

'MY GOAL IS TO STAY SLIM AND HEALTHY INTO MY 50s'

Tracy Bridgett, 49
Senior manager
Height 1.75m (5ft 9in)

Before	After
79kg (12st 5½lb)	70kg (11st ½lb)
Dress size 16	Dress size 12

WEIGHT LOST 9KG (1ST 5LB)

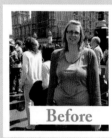

Before

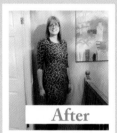

After

I was always very skinny as a child and young woman and I found I could eat whatever I wanted without gaining weight. After having my children and hitting 35, the number on the scales started to creep up and the pounds stayed on. When I lost my mum I comfort ate and put on even more weight. When my clothes reached a size 16 I felt frumpy — that's when I decided I needed to do something about my weight gain.

I began running regularly, something that I had not done for years. To help me get going I bought an interval-training app on my smartphone that started off with very short runs mixed with walking. Eventually, following the app, I slowly increased my time spent running and decreased my time spent walking, until I was running 10K (6 miles) comfortably.

I started to feel fantastic. Running really changed the shape of my body. Many people say I look as if I've lost much more weight than I have and I'm sure that's thanks to my toned physique.

I have bought lots of gorgeous new clothes for work and love showing off my new figure. My goal is to stay slim and healthy into my 50s.

After losing weight I now run much more seriously, usually two to three times per week. I'm planning to run a half-marathon next. I also try to walk and use the stairs whenever possible and even running for my train is easy if I'm late!

HOW TRACY DID IT

Training tip: 'I find listening to upbeat, high tempo music keeps me going on a run. Setting up a playlist with running tracks on saves skipping through songs that aren't right mid-run.'

Motivation tip: 'Following beginners' running apps available to download on smartphones is a great way to get started and many are free.'

'I RAN MY WAY INTO A SIZE 12 WEDDING DRESS'

Karen Reeve, 28
PA
Height 1.7m (5ft 7in)

Before	After
86kg (13st 8lb)	64kg (10st 1lb)
Dress size 18/20	Dress size 12

WEIGHT LOST 22KG (3ST 7LB)

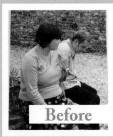

Before

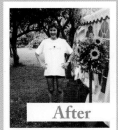

After

If someone had told me, as I sat crying about the way I looked, that in less than 12 months I'd be 22kg (3st 7lb) slimmer, I wouldn't have believed them. A hideous photo of me taken at my partner Nick's 30th birthday prompted me to get fit. I didn't have the money for a gym, so I opted for running. The day I promised myself I'd start, a storm was raging but I set off regardless. I had to combine small amounts of running with walking because I was so unfit but, despite the weather, it was really exhilarating and I've never looked back.

Nick had proposed to me a short time before I started running, so I used the wedding as an incentive to keep up my new fitness and healthy-eating regime. I lost the weight easily, and each dress fitting reminded me of how far I'd come, making me all the more determined to succeed. By the time I got married, I was overjoyed that I was going to be a slim bride.

I'd always said I was going to go for a run on my wedding day, and I meant it. That morning, I leaped out of bed and opened the presents Nick had given me the night before. My favourite was a personalised T-shirt with a twist! On one side it said the name of our church and our wedding date, and on the reverse it said 'bride'. I ran only 5K (3 miles) that day but I felt really elated. I still smile when I think of all the congratulatory beeps from passing drivers as they read my T-shirt! At the reception Nick made a speech and held up the T-shirt, saying, 'Karen was really determined to go for a run this morning, so I made her this.' It was lovely and everyone gave me a round of applause.

I'm still totally passionate about running and feel I owe a lot to it. Anyone who says they can't run is wrong – just look at me!

HOW KAREN DID IT

Training tip: 'Follow a training programme – and stick to it. I typed mine up and loved crossing through every run once I'd finished it.'
Motivation tip: 'Give yourself rewards. I had a special nutty cereal that I ate after my weekly 21K (13-mile) route. I really looked forward to it.'

'I FEEL LIKE I CAN CONQUER THE WORLD!'

Louise Carsley-Black, 42
International banker
Height 1.63m (5ft 4in)

Before	After
121kg (19st 1lb)	75kg (11st 11½lb)
Dress size 18	Dress size 8/10

WEIGHT LOST 46KG (7ST 3½LB)

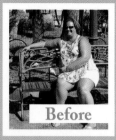

Before

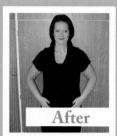

After

I had been overweight for over 25 years before I made the conscious decision to make a change. From the age of 16 when leaving school and starting work, my weight just crept up and up. The final straw came on holiday in Spain with my husband of only two years – I couldn't stand the heat and couldn't even go for a walk along the beach. I knew it was time to take action.

I decided to join my local slimming group and lost 46kg (7st 3lb) in 18 months through eating healthy, balanced meals and gradually increasing my activity levels. As I lost weight I started running, having never run before in my life, and signed up to run a 10K (6 mile) race in aid of the British Heart Foundation. At first I went at completely my own pace, and gradually tried to go further each time. The small increments soon added up and I managed to reach the distance before the day of the race. After that I was able to work on improving my time.

Currently I am aiming to achieve a time of less than 45 minutes for a 10K (6 mile) run.

My life has improved beyond compare. I have just started a new job after 26 years working for the same company – I would never have had the confidence to even attend an interview before. My life is already a million light-years away from where I was just 12 months ago. I feel like I can conquer the world!

HOW LOUISE DID IT
Training tip: 'I have a very supportive family and find running with my son a great way for us to spend time together. We both enjoy it and it's a bonus that we can keep fit at the same time.'
Motivation tip: 'Running for charity was a huge pull for me, knowing I am running for a special cause makes the training and race itself even more special.'

'I HAVE SO MUCH MORE CONFIDENCE'

Lorna Needham, 31
Full-time mum
Height 1.65m (5ft 5in)

Before	After
96kg (15st 2½lb)	64kg (10st 2½lb)
Dress size 22	Dress size 10

WEIGHT LOST 32KG (5ST)

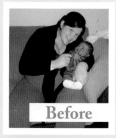

Before

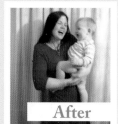

After

I had always been the 'bigger one' at school and in the family. This continued into adulthood and I went on to gain a lot of weight during my first pregnancy. I lost some weight after that but following my third pregnancy I had a condition that meant I was on crutches. Despite not being able to get around, I ate what I wanted and it turned into a vicious cycle – the bigger I got the less able I was to move, and the more I ate.

Being a mum of three, I found a local gym to join which also had a crèche. It only opened an hour a day and so I booked it each week, giving me an incentive to go and take that time to improve my fitness. I used the treadmill and started off slowly, gradually increasing the length and speed when I felt comfortable. My fitness soon improved and I found I could do more and more each week.

Now I try to do two weekly 10K (6 mile) runs on the treadmill.

Before I was very unfit and could not join in family activities with my children, always watching longingly from the sidelines. I got out of breath climbing the stairs and needed to sit down when I got to the top. I had no confidence at all and made up excuses as to why I couldn't go out.

Now I am 32kg (5st) lighter and can run up the stairs, enjoy walks, have the confidence to have photographs taken and shop for clothes. The children are always on the go and it feels fantastic knowing I can keep up with them now. I have so much more confidence.

HOW LORNA DID IT

Training tip: 'I like to race against myself and try to beat my own personal best time or distance. It's amazing how much more you can do when you push yourself that tiny bit.'

Motivation tip: 'Pre-planning my runs at the start of the week keeps me on track. That way I know to keep that time free and can stick to my schedule more easily.'

'I CAN DO MUCH MORE WITH MY BODY THAN BEFORE'

Laura Barnes, 26
Web project leader
Height 1.63m (5ft 4in)

Before	After
89kg (14st)	54kg (8st 7lb)
Dress size 18	Dress size 8/10

WEIGHT LOST 35KG (5ST 7LB)

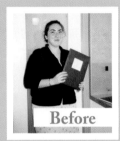
Before

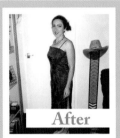
After

I put on a lot of weight at university by feasting on tubs of ice cream and drinking lots of gin and tonics, but I found it hard to motivate myself to change my habits and get fit. Although I always knew running would be a brilliant way of losing weight, I felt apprehensive about trying it as I'd always failed at it in the past. I also really worried about people seeing the colour my face went on a run. But then a truly awful photo of me looking podgy-faced and piggy-eyed finally motivated me to start losing weight.

After about 13kg (2st) had come off, I entered a 5K (3-mile) race with three friends – I loved the fact that it was an all-women run because it felt really non-competitive. Having something like that looming meant I had to start training, so I set off with a friend, doing just 30 seconds at a time with lots of walking in between. We were amazed at how fast we built up to running 8K (5 miles), and even had enough puff left to talk the whole time! I found race day terrifying, but the four of us ran together until competition got the better of us and I won the sprint for the finish line!

Running got me fitter than anything else I'd ever tried, and helped me lose more weight than I'd ever thought possible – a total of 35kg (5st 7lb). My appearance changed so much that the compliments started to flood in and even my own mum once walked past me without recognising me!

The experience also completely transformed my view of what I'm capable of. Something I feared has now become something I love. I even keep my race medal on view to remind me of my achievements. I've realised I can do much more with my body than before. Now, instead of sitting at work feeling big and miserable, I sit there itching to get outside and run.

HOW LAURA DID IT
Training tip: 'I don't tell myself I have to run for a certain time or distance – sometimes I literally just go round the block, which takes only 4 minutes.'
Motivation tip: 'Running along chatting with a friend made even 6.5K (4-mile) runs fun and helped them to pass more quickly.'

'RUNNING IS GOOD FOR BODY AND SOUL'

Shonagh Woods, 34
Marketing manager
Height 1.68m (5ft 6in)

	Before	After
	79kg (12st 6lb)	60kg (9st 6lb)
	Dress size 14/16	Dress size 10

WEIGHT LOST 19KG (3ST)

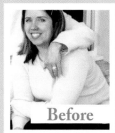
Before

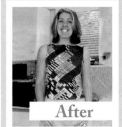
After

When I started bulging out of my size 14 clothes but couldn't bear to buy a size 16, I knew I had to do something about my weight. I felt as if the real me was hiding inside the body of a fat person and couldn't get out. Things changed when I got engaged and realised I had to lose the weight fast for my wedding. I simply couldn't bear the idea of being a fat bride, and the thought of my future children looking at my fat wedding photos filled me with horror.

I wasn't sure where to start until my best friend bought me a brilliant book on running for Christmas. I'd always thought of running as boring but the book really inspired me. There was a long, straight road where I lived, and I'd set off running along it for 5 minutes then run back for five.

When I was able to run for 10 minutes out and 10 back, I hopped in the car to measure the distance and was ecstatic to find I could run 3K (2 miles)! I found the running was not only making me lose weight – about 3kg (7lb) a month – but was good for my soul, too. I started feeling I was back in control of my life again. Muscles were appearing in my legs and along the sides of my stomach where I'd never known they existed, and my jeans became too big.

On my wedding day I was 13kg (2st) lighter and felt brilliant – there wasn't a single photo I didn't like. But things have got even better since. I went on to run my first half-marathon (21K/13.1miles) and at 60kg (9st 6lb) I'm now down to my slimmest ever. I also feel amazingly positive about other things in life that I might once have doubted I could do, be or say. Because I started from scratch and transformed myself into a runner, I now believe I can achieve whatever I want.

HOW SHONAGH DID IT
Training tip: 'Don't think you can't run – just get yourself a good pair of trainers and then set off really slowly.'
Motivation tip: 'Realise what running can do for your mind. I always come back from a run feeling a lot less stressed, full of ideas and with solutions to my problems.'

'MY FITNESS LEVELS IMPROVED SO QUICKLY'

Hannah Smith, 34
Learning and development consultant
Height 1.7m (5ft 7in)

Before	After
103kg (16st 3½lb)	75kg (11st 12½lb)
Dress size 22	Dress size 12

WEIGHT LOST 28KG (4ST 5LB)

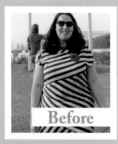

Before

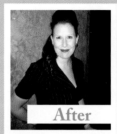

After

My weight was constantly up and down as a teenager although I slimmed down in my late teens. I then gained a lot of weight back in my early 20s, which I later lost by attending slimming classes and then by taking up running. After putting back on more weight than I felt comfortable with, I started to feel really low. A big part of that was down to being unfit and unable to do what I wanted to do.

My friend had been doing lots of running and was training to do the London Marathon; talking to her about it made me remember how much I used to enjoy running in my younger years. I found myself wishing I could run again but thought it would be just too hard at the weight I had got to, and too much strain on my joints.

I had been overweight for about five years before I made the conscious decision to get slim. I joined Slimming World and as I started to lose weight I started running again. I started out by walking and then built in running over time; setting myself distance targets to aim for kept me on track to start with, particularly when it was difficult to exercise. As I got more comfortable I built variety into my exercise routine with strength-based exercise as well as just running.

When I first started I could only run for a couple of minutes at a time, but in a few months I was able to run further and further. My fitness levels improved so quickly. Now I can run a 21K (13.1 mile) half-marathon!

HOW HANNAH DID IT
Training tip: 'I found that setting incremental targets was the most effective way to keep going. Signing up to a variety of races and telling people about them also really motivated me.'
Motivation tip: 'If you've got a friend who also loves running, try and encourage each other to keep going and try new things.'

'I THOUGHT I WAS DESTINED TO BE FAT FOR EVER'

Julie McWhirr, 27
Investment banker
Height 1.63m (5ft 4in)

Before	After
94kg (14st 11lb)	66kg (10st 6lb)
Dress size 20	Dress size 12

WEIGHT LOST 28KG (4ST 5LB)

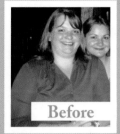

Before

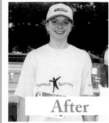

After

The crunch came when I was out shopping for a special outfit. I'd convinced myself I looked OK in the size 20 dress I was trying on, until I found myself in front of the communal mirror next to a size 10 girl trying on the same dress! I realized then that I had to do something about the ridiculous amount of weight I'd put on, so when a friend joined Weight Watchers, I followed suit. After I'd lost the first 4.5kg (10lb), I started to exercise gently by walking on a treadmill. I'm a determined person with lots of willpower, so I stuck at it until I could gradually turn up the speed and start running. After each run, I started to feel a high I'd never experienced before. And the more weight I lost, the more confidence I had to do new things, like join an all-women running club (called The Epsom Allsorts because it's a real mix of people, from girls to grandmas!).

The weight kept falling off steadily, while the running started to tone me. I was also developing collarbones – it's such a novelty to have them there!

But the best thing about running was that it kept me positive and gave me a non-weight-related goal that stopped the weigh-in at Weight Watchers dictating my whole mood for the week. In fact, by the time I'd reached my goal weight of 66kg (10st 6lb), I had another, more important goal in mind – to run a half-marathon (21K/13.1 miles).

The race was incredible! I loved every minute of it and kept slowing down because I wanted it to last longer. I always thought I was destined to be fat for the rest of my life – these days, I often walk past shop windows and don't recognize myself. And I know that by keeping on running, I'll stay this way for good.

HOW JULIE DID IT

Motivation tip: 'If I ever lack motivation, I ask my partner Ian to give me three good reasons why I should go for a run. By the time he's listed them, I'm up off the sofa and out of the front door.'

Eating tip: 'Even if you're trying to lose weight, you do need to eat enough to give you the energy to run. Don't expect to go out and run for miles on a diet of salad and apples alone.'

DO YOU WANT TO WAKE UP HAPPY EVERY DAY AND BOUNCE THROUGH LIFE WITH A PERMANENT SMILE ON YOUR FACE? ALL IT TAKES TO FEEL THIS GOOD IS SOMETHING THAT GETS YOUR MIND AS FIT AS YOUR BODY – WE RECOMMEND A REGULAR DOSE OF RUNNING ...

3. GET HAPPY

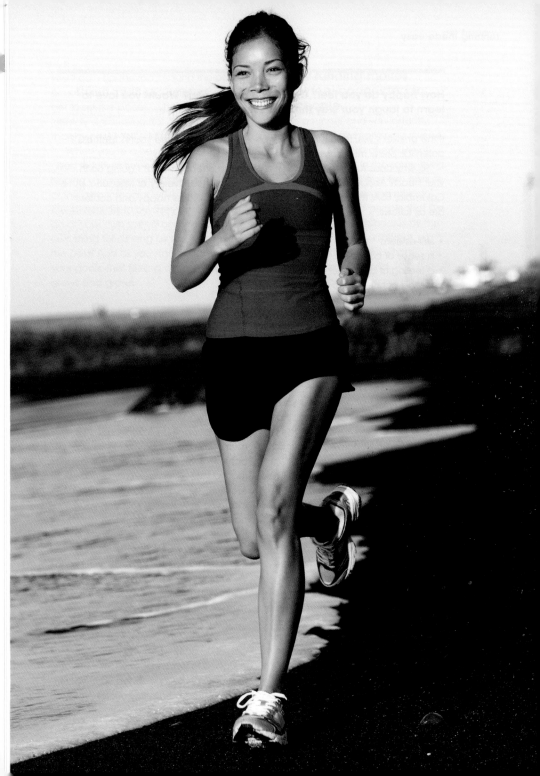

'HOW RUNNING MAKES ME FEEL'

WE CHALLENGED THESE RUNNERS TO CAPTURE IN WORDS THE MOOD-BOOSTING, GRIN-INDUCING POWER OF RUNNING ...

'Running makes me feel free. **This is the time I can be me,** no pretending or trying to measure up to anyone else's expectations. I run only against myself. Every week when I go out for my long run I surprise myself. How is it that this girl who hated running at school can now run comfortably for 2 hours? I've started doing interval training and love those little bursts of speed too. Running first thing on a summer morning is glorious and even on a cold dark one it is pretty good: getting to work feeling energized.'
Penny Rance, 33, online co-ordinator, Surrey

'I love running because wherever you are in the world, and however you felt before you went for a run, it always has the same effect. Once you've been running, **you feel like a different and better person.** The problem that was nagging away at you has been solved. The sluggishness brought on by jet lag has evaporated, the anger and irritation left behind. Running – always the solution, never the problem.'
Marcus Leaver, 33, CEO, London

'Running, particularly off-road, makes me feel alive. Listening to the birds and feeling the wind in my hair and the changing ground underfoot helps me to lose myself in the moment and de-stress. My long runs in particular give me a real sense of achievement. **I feel good about myself after running, even if I come home soaked with sweat or rain and with aching legs.** As event director of the Parkrun in Croydon's Lloyd Park, I've also been in a great position to see hundreds of people use running to improve their fitness and health. I've been delighted to watch families happily running together – including teenagers! – and sharing each others' achievements.'
Debra Bourne, 46, veterinary surgeon, London

'Running is my "secret weapon" – it gave me the confidence to write for the school newspaper and try out for the hockey team when I was young, and **it continues to make me feel powerful, free and fearless** to this day. The biggest thing I've learned from running over 53 years of doing it, is that it's given me just about everything in my life that matters – my health, my career, my husband ... but most of all, it has given me myself. Also, any day you can run makes the day somehow worthwhile even when everything else may not be so good.'
Kathrine Switzer, 67, the first woman to officially run what was then the all-male Boston Marathon, and author of *Marathon Woman*

'I've been amazed by how much better I feel for running after the birth of my son. Around the time he turned one, I gingerly donned my trainers and set off at tortoise pace. Now I run about three times a week once he's in bed. **Even when I'm tired, it picks me up,** makes me feel better about my body shape and reminds me I'm still my own person as well as a mum!'
Jill Hopper, 38, journalist, London

'Running gives me a terrific **sense of achievement** and makes me feel alive, even when my lungs are straining and my legs are exhausted.'
Dan Waugh, 30, corporate affairs manager, London

'I adore the feeling of nervous excitement that I get at the start of a marathon, in fact it's rather addictive! I'd already done 15 marathons when I decided to celebrate the Olympics coming to London by running 2,012 miles in 2012. Only problem was, I soon had to search for another goal as I'd already reached that total by May! **In the end I ran 21 marathons and the sense of achievement was immense.** Running has given me incredible self-belief and has helped me become the person I always wanted to be.'
Penny Lovegrove, 65, pensioner, Bouth, The Lake District

'Running is **like going into your own private room.** I do my best thinking when I'm running because it really helps clear my mind.'
Alan Nurse, 34, solicitor, London

'The joy of being alive in the small hours of a sparkling, clear morning, and running amid idyllic landscapes of cool green forests, pastoral valleys, mountain scenery and glistening coastlines is the main reason I love running as much as I do.'
Ginette Flockton, 55, teacher, Cape Town, South Africa

'When I moved from South Africa to Winnipeg in Canada, which gets down to an unbelievable -40˚C (-40˚F), running outside in the winter months didn't seem like an option! However, while running in a windowless basement gym, I was eventually persuaded by a concerned fellow runner to ditch running on the dreadmill (!) and give outdoor running a go. On my first outing **I felt sheer joy** as I raced across the frozen, snow-covered Assiniboine River. Now I run every day in the most beautiful place I've ever run in!'
Bridget Robinson, 46, project manager, Winnipeg, Canada

WALT DISNEY ONCE SAID, 'IF YOU CAN DREAM IT, YOU CAN DO IT!' THIS CHAPTER IS YOUR CHANCE TO DREAM – AND ACHIEVE ANY GOAL YOU'VE SET YOUR HEART ON ...

4. GET SET FOR SUCCESS

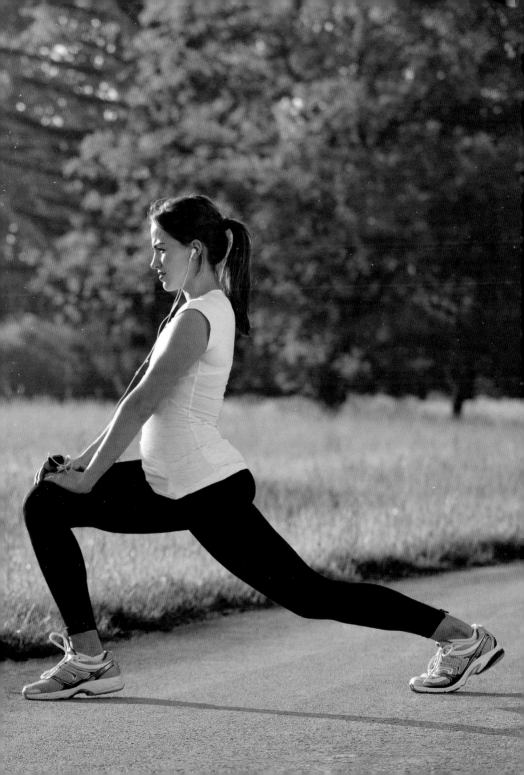

Rather like window-shopping, when you're not actually intending to buy anything and just want to see what's out there, running along without any real purpose can be great fun. But running with a goal in mind can be even better – just as window-shopping becomes more exciting when you spot your perfect pair of designer shoes and know you'll do anything to afford them. Another reason why having something to aim for is important is that experts say 'progressively achieving worthwhile goals' can actually make you happy. So prepare to feel fantastic, because running is unbeatable at providing you with limitless goal-setting opportunities. It's progressive, too, as the training plans you to follow (see Chapters 6 and 8) will help you achieve these goals one step at a time. And, of course, it goes without saying that these goals are incredibly worthwhile – achieving them will turbo-boost your vitality, your health, your self-image and your mood.

SIX STEPS TO SUCCESS

How do you go about reaching your goals? It's not as difficult as you may have feared. Basically, you can break it all down into six simple steps:

1. Choose your goal

When you're casting about for a goal, remember that, as one author once put it, 'Goals are dreams with deadlines.' Goal-setting simply involves finding out what your dreams really are – and then setting about making them happen within a set time frame.

Let's do some dreaming right now. First take a look at the Why I Want To Get Fit list (see opposite), which gives you some ideas to get you started, plus space to add your own at the bottom of the page. Then, for the next five minutes, close your eyes and dream the impossible dream, which, we promise, will become the possible dream sooner than you think. How would you like to look in six months' time? How would you like to feel? What would you like to have accomplished? The kind of goal you should be thinking of should really excite you and give you butterflies in your stomach and shivers down your spine.

Dare to dream big – and don't think to yourself – and don't think to yourself, 'I'd love to run a 5K (3 mile) race but I'll have to wait until I'm slimmer/fitter/ have more time/have given up smoking', as by doing that you're placing limits on what you can achieve.

WHY I WANT TO GET FIT

▶▶▶

▶▶ I want to love myself more, but have less of me to love.

▶▶ I want to be able to put all my photos in my albums – not just the ones where my double chin isn't showing.

▶▶ I want people to say, 'You're looking well' and know that they really mean, 'Wow, you've lost weight!'

▶▶ I want to feel happier.

▶▶ I want to be able to buy clothes in a smaller size.

▶▶ I want to keep up with my hyperactive kids.

▶▶ I want to be able to do a 5K (3 mile) fun run with my friends – and actually have fun doing it.

▶▶ I want to quit smoking.

▶▶ I want to attend my school reunion and show everyone how amazing I look.

▶▶ I want to shop for head-turning clothes rather than live in baggy tracksuit bottoms and sloppy jumpers.

▶▶ I want to be able to race up stairs and escalators without breaking into a sweat.

▶▶ I want to feel young again.

▶▶ I want to run a race in a fairy outfit.

▶▶ I want to take my stress out on the street, not on my partner or my dog.

▶▶ I want to send my self-esteem rocketing.

▶▶ I want to boost my chances of getting a telegram from the Queen on my 100th birthday.

▶▶ I want to banish my pot belly for good and stop letting out notches on my belt.

▶▶ I want to be smelling the daisies when I'm old – not pushing them up.

▶▶ I want to boost my mood – without reaching for the biscuits.

▶▶ I want to win medals without joining the army.

▶▶ I want to spend quality time getting to know the real me.

▶▶ I want to _____

▶▶ I want to _____

▶▶ I want to _____

▶▶ I want to _____

▶▶ I want to _____

▶▶ I want to _____

Just as no one can make you feel inferior without your consent (as the USA First Lady Eleanor Roosevelt famously said), no one can put limits on what you can achieve without your permission either. 'I now realize the limits I set for myself were just excuses and that I can do anything, and go as far as I want to go,' says Catherine Mokwena, 41, a South African runner who ran the New York City Marathon with an artificial leg.

So even if you're really overweight, desperately out of shape, manically busy and a 20-a-day smoker, just set your goal and leave worrying about how you're going to achieve it to us! Now write your long-term dream goal into your Mission Statement, which you'll find on page 47.

2. Make sure it's a SMART goal

SMART goals are successful goals. The acronym SMART stands for:

Specific Being very precise about what you want to achieve will give you something tangible to aim for – an example of a specific goal is saying, 'I want to run a 5K (3 mile) race in three months' time dressed as a superhero.' An example of a non-specific goal would simply be saying, 'I want to get fit.'

Measurable This will enable you to know when you've succeeded – which means it's time to celebrate! A good example of a measurable goal would be saying, 'I want to be 13kg (2st) lighter a year from now and be able to fit into my favourite pair of jeans.'

Achievable Be honest with yourself about your abilities and don't set yourself up for failure by deciding on goals that are totally out of reach (but don't let this stop you dreaming big!). So, while aiming to win your first-ever race may be unrealistic, vowing to come in the top half of the field may be well within your grasp.

Reward-orientated Plan an 'I-deserve-this' treat for every time you achieve your goals to reinforce your good behaviour and encourage you to keep going.

Time-framed Giving yourself a deadline will provide a sense of urgency – and make you all the more likely to succeed.

3. Break it into bite-sized chunks

Next, set a date for when you want to achieve your goal by and write it into your Mission Statement (see page 47). Then chop it into easily digestible (and do-able) chunks. Breaking down a long-term goal into lots of short-term goals you know you're capable of achieving is the key to success. This is often tricky, so you'll be relieved we've already done all the hard work and set out a ten-week step-by-step programme called The 60-Second-Secret Plan for you to follow (see Chapter 6).

4. Work out your rewards

Now it's time for the fun part! Look at the Daily Rewards, Weekly Treats and Ultimate Indulgences (see opposite) for some ideas on how you can reward yourself for all your hard work and commitment.

DAILY REWARDS

▶▶ Read a magazine for half an hour.

▶▶ Savour an ice-cold beer.

▶▶ Wallow in the bath.

▶▶ Eat a healthy treat such as melon, strawberries, lychees or passion fruit.

▶▶ Snooze on the sofa for 30 minutes.

▶▶ Spend 10 minutes relaxing in your garden.

▶▶ Read a chapter of a great novel.

▶▶ Phone a friend for a chat.

▶▶ Watch an episode from your favourite box set.

▶▶ Spend 10 minutes in the sauna or steam room at your gym.

WEEKLY TREATS

▶▶ Buy a figure-flattering piece of fit kit.

▶▶ Subscribe to a health or fitness magazine, such as *Runner's World* or *Women's* or *Men's Running*.

▶▶ Buy a new book.

▶▶ Have a pampering home spa session in your bathroom.

▶▶ Go out for a slap-up meal.

▶▶ Go to see a great new film.

▶▶ Treat yourself to a healthy brunch.

▶▶ Have a night out on the town.

▶▶ Download a new track from iTunes.

▶▶ Get that lipstick/nail colour/pair headphones you've had your eye on.

▶▶ Buy a big bunch of fresh flowers.

▶▶ Spend an evening in front of the fire with a bottle of good wine.

▶▶ Laugh yourself silly at a comedy club.

▶▶ Have a date night with your partner.

▶▶ Go and see some live music.

ULTIMATE INDULGENCES

▶▶ Buy that amazing outfit you've been coveting.

▶▶ Do something adrenalin-fuelled like skydiving or bungee jumping.

▶▶ Go to the ballet, opera or a classical concert.

▶▶ Sign up for a course in something you've always dreamed of doing: scuba diving, wine tasting, yoga or Indian head massage.

▶▶ Treat yourself to a gym membership.

▶▶ Have a new haircut.

▶▶ Go to a glamorous sporting event such as a day at the races, a grand prix or a football final.

▶▶ Indulge yourself with a course of facials, manicures or massages.

▶▶ Buy a pair of designer shoes.

▶▶ Book a romantic weekend break or exotic holiday.

POTENTIAL PENALTIES

✖ No TV for a week.

✖ Ban yourself from eating your favourite food for a month.

✖ Postpone that haircut/root retouching you know you need.

✖ No alcohol for a month.

✖ Do one of those grim household tasks you've been putting off, like clearing out the plughole in the shower, or hoovering behind the sofa.

5. Write it down

Along with this book, your daily diary (and your trainers!), your pen is your greatest ally in reaching your goal. Use it to complete the rest of your Mission Statement, to fill in the results of the fitness tests in Chapter 5 and to schedule in each of The 60-Second-Secret Plan sessions (see Chapter 6) in your diary so you'll stick to your programme, stay focused and avoid getting side-tracked.

How's this for an amazing story that proves the power of the pen? In a study of students who'd recently graduated from Yale, only 3% said they'd written down specific goals for what they hoped to achieve in the future. Years later, when the graduates were surveyed again, the 3% who'd written down their goals had not only achieved most of what they'd hoped for, but their net worth equalled that of the other 97% combined. Worth trying for yourself, don't you think?

6. Get going!

But not before you've done the four fabulous fitness tests in the next chapter. However, if you feel you really can't wait to get started, turn to page 66 to sneak a look at what the amazing 60-Second-Secret Plan has in store for you ...

MY MISSION STATEMENT

▶▶▶

I, _____**(name)**, being of sound mind, and slightly less sound body, do solemnly declare that I have decided to commit myself to getting fit. My **long-term dream goal** is to _____

_____,

which I aim to achieve by _____**(date)**. I have chosen this goal because (choose two of the **reasons** you ticked or wrote in your Why I Want To Get Fit list on page 43)

1._____

2._____

In order to achieve this long-term dream goal, I hereby commit myself to sticking faithfully to my short-term goals in The 60-Second-Secret Plan.

I promise, every single time I complete a session from the plan, to **celebrate** by treating myself with a **Daily Reward** from the list on page 45. And at the end of every week that I've stuck to the programme, I'll celebrate by rewarding myself with _____ (choose a **Weekly Treat** from the list on page 45). After successfully completing the programme, I'll celebrate by spoiling myself with _____

_____ (choose an **Ultimate Indulgence** from the list). I also promise faithfully to read this Mission Statement daily to remind myself of my goal (and my rewards!).

Today's date_____

Date I will have completed my short-term goals by (ten weeks' time)

_____

However, if I fail to complete The 60-Second-Secret Plan (odd lapses don't count!), I promise to_____

(insert a penalty from the **Potential Penalties** list on page 45).

TOP TIP Photocopy this Mission Statement and keep a copy in your wallet, your daily diary or Filofax and your gym bag. Stick a copy of it on your fridge door, next to your bathroom mirror or on your computer and look at it frequently to remind yourself of what you're determined to achieve. As Martin Luther King Jr said, 'I have a dream ...' Remember, you have one, too, now – all you have to do is go out and make it come true.

'WHY I RUN'

HERE'S WHY THESE PEOPLE CHOSE RUNNING AS THEIR GOAL – AND WHY THEY'RE STILL AT IT, AND LOVING IT, YEARS LATER . . .

'Running's just awesome. Surfers have an expression, 'Only a surfer knows the feeling,' and it's the same with running. You can't describe it, you just have to feel it. It's **such a good feeling** when you're running tall and relaxed and your legs are just flowing through beneath you.'
Rob Banister, 24, facilities manager, Sydney, Australia

'In early 2002 I discovered **I had very high cholesterol levels and decided to change my diet radically.** As a result of eating more healthily and running, I've lost about 25.5kg (4st) and dropped from over 95.5kg (15st) to 70kg (11st), which is the weight I was when I started university. The more weight I lost, the more enjoyable running felt, until it became a pleasure in its own right. I'm amazed when I look back and realize that going for a run now at my old weight would be the equivalent of running with a young child sitting on my back!'
Duncan Edwards, 49, president and CEO, Hearst Magazines International, London

'I have traumatic memories of cross-country races when all the other kids ran like aspiring athletes while I puffed along unhappily at the back, amazed that their lungs weren't on the verge of exploding from the lack of oxygen. Now that I'm running again 20 years later, I'm surprised it's so effortless – except, that is, when those dreaded hills loom and the emotions of a ten-year-old come flooding back into my 30-something being. I feel totally breathless, utterly hopeless and wretchedly miserable! And then I know why I run. It's because **it makes me feel young again!'**
Lize Lombard, lawyer, 32, Wimbledon

'**I run to keep fit and to relax,** and because I think a great deal when I'm running – I plan the day and wonder whom I'm going to drive crazy in the magazine business. During the week I live in London and follow the same running routine two or three times a week. I get up early and run a circuit that always passes the Houses of Parliament, where I check the time on Big Ben, before heading home again. Although as I get older I really have to discipline myself to do it, and sometimes it feels more like 30 miles than five or six, it makes me feel fresh, and sets me up for the day.'
Terry Mansfield CBE, 75, consultant, The Hearst Corporation, London

'I started running as part of a plan to get fitter, but now running is about more than just the exercise. **For me, it's about spending time alone,** outside, taking in the sights and sounds. Rather than punishing myself for stopping to catch my breath, I enjoy stopping to hear the birds or to admire a pretty front garden.'
Sophie Easton, 33, crime scene examiner for the Metropolitan Police, Surrey

'I run for fun. I sometimes compete in races, but I don't ever want running to become a chore. I like choosing where and how far I run, rather than sticking to a training plan. As a personal trainer, I really enjoy mixing up my exercise routine to include lots of different activities. Throughout this, running has always been a constant. **Running is free, you can do it anywhere, and you will always feel better for it afterwards!'**
Chloe Bowler, 33, personal trainer, London

'On Saturday mornings I go running in the woods near my home. All I can hear is my breath and the crunching of snow. I'm constantly watching for moose that wander down from the hills when it gets cold. I'm a little more relaxed than when I run here in the summer, because the bears and their cubs are hibernating now. At about 10K (6 miles), I usually decide that it's time to head back. In the last few **minutes of every run I do, I take time to give thanks for the good things in my life** – the air in my lungs, the beauty I get to behold, the ability to love something such as running so much that my heart swells when I just think about it.'
Michael K Deems Jr, 26, army officer, Fairbanks, Alaska, USA

'I run because even though I struggle with it, I know it's the absolute best thing I can do for my fitness. **I've never felt fitter than when I trained for a marathon.** Going for a bike ride or playing football just doesn't give you the same feeling. So I soldier on with it, even though I complain bitterly before every run!'
Adam Makepeace, 31, solicitor, London

'My wife always said she fell in love with me because **I had such good legs** – something I attribute to all the athletics I did at university. Reason enough, then, I thought, to carry on running once I left university. And so for 40 years I've gone for a 20-minute run after work each day. At 75, I'm proud to say I can still fit into the blazer I wore when I first met my wife!'
Anthony Jackson, 75, law student, Pretoria, South Africa

ARE YOU READY TO GO ON A VOYAGE
OF SELF-DISCOVERY? WANT TO KNOW
THE REAL YOU AND WHAT YOU'RE
CAPABLE OF? WE'VE SELECTED FOUR
KEY FITNESS TESTS AND TURNED
THEM INTO HIGHLY MOTIVATIONAL
TOOLS YOU CAN USE TO TRACK YOUR
PROGRESS AND KEEP YOU INSPIRED.
YOUR FIRST STEP TO A FITTER,
MORE FABULOUS YOU STARTS
RIGHT HERE ...

5. GET TO KNOW YOURSELF

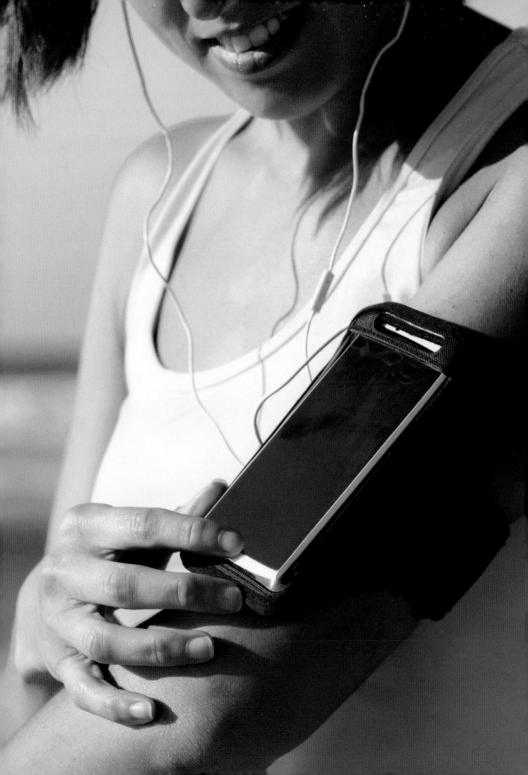

It's time to get cracking! You've completed your Mission Statement and now you need to establish how fit you are so you can monitor your progress as you shape up. Nothing will be more motivating than noting how your heartbeat slows as your fitness improves, watching those inches melt off, charting your weight loss as you gradually slim down and seeing your body-fat levels dropping.

DO I HAVE TO DO ALL THE TESTS?

No, but the more you do, the more you'll be able to bask in the glow of satisfaction that comes from knowing you're building a better, stronger, healthier body. Regularly doing these tests means you'll almost always have positive, concrete evidence of how much good your running programme is doing you.

The reason we've given you four to do is that even if you aren't quite as successful as you'd hoped in one area, such as weight loss, you'll still be able to see the real improvements you've made in other areas, such as your measurements. If you rely only on your scales to keep you motivated, you may be tempted to throw in the towel if there hasn't been any evidence of weight loss. However, if you also take your measurements, you'll notice that you've lost inches and can fit into your clothes more easily. Remember, changes in shape are just as important, healthwise, as weight loss. Reason enough to stick with the programme until you do lose some weight? You bet!

HOW SHOULD I DO THESE TESTS?

To make sure these tests are as accurate as possible, do them at the same time of day (evening is best for monitoring your body-fat percentage, morning is best for the other three), wearing the same kind of clothing. Repeat them as directed to give you a clear idea of just how well you're doing. And don't forget to make a note in your diary to remind yourself to do them regularly.

YOUR SELF-TEST KIT

- **Pen**

- **Pencil**

- **Tape measure**

- **Diary** (so you can note when you'll need to do the tests in the weeks and months to come)

- **Scales** (preferably those that can measure body-fat composition)

- **Watch** that can time seconds.

- **Gym membership** or personal trainer (for body-fat percentage monitoring purposes – this is entirely optional!)

ALL ABOUT YOU: 4 FABULOUS FITNESS TESTS

TEST 1: RESTING HEART RATE

WHAT YOU'LL NEED
- Watch
- Pen

WHY DO IT?
Measuring your heart rate (or pulse) when you're at rest is a good way to assess your cardiovascular fitness because the stronger your heart is, the fewer times a minute it has to pump to send blood around your body.

WHAT TO DO
Do this test first thing in the morning so the results won't be affected by physical activities or stress. And avoid taking stimulants such as caffeine or nicotine before doing it.

Take your pulse at your wrist for 15 seconds, using your finger. Now multiply the number of heartbeats you counted by four to get your heart rate in beats per minute (bpm). If this figure is over 100, visit your GP as soon as you can as this may mean you have an abnormal heart rhythm that could potentially be dangerous.

WHAT IT ALL MEANS
If you're running regularly, you can expect your resting heart rate to drop by one or two beats per minute every one to two weeks. If you've trained well, after six months you could be looking at a drop of between 10bpm and 15bpm. However, your heart rate will only drop a maximum of 20 beats.

MY RESTING HEART RATE		
	Date / time	Resting heart rate in beats per minute
Today		
After 1 week		
After 2 weeks		
After 3 weeks		
After 4 weeks		
After 5 weeks		
After 6 weeks		
After 7 weeks		
After 8 weeks		
After 9 weeks		
After 10 weeks		
After 3 months		
After 4 months		
After 5 months		
After 6 months		

TEST 2: MEASUREMENTS

WHAT YOU'LL NEED

- Tape measure
- Pen

WHY DO IT?

By measuring different parts of your body, you'll be able to keep track of how you're firming up and the way your body is changing as the fat melts away. Mind you, your declining bank balance as you regularly have to buy new clothes in smaller sizes will also be a brilliant indicator of how well you're doing!

Your waist measurement is probably the most important of the five measurements to focus on, as it can be a very valuable way to assess your health risks. This is because scientists now know that where you carry your extra weight can have a big impact on your health.

Pear-shaped people who have smaller waists and tend to carry extra weight on their hips and thighs are healthier than apple-shaped people who carry extra weight around their stomach. This is because fat comes in different types (yes, really!), and the type that is stored on the lower body is known as 'subcutaneous' and poses less of a health risk.

Fat that is stored deep within the abdomen, however, is known as 'visceral' and scientists now know it pumps out hormones and other substances that can lead to a range of health problems (see 'What it all means').

WHAT TO DO

Use the tape measure to take the measurements (in either inches or centimetres) of the following parts of your body – remember that for you to chart your progress accurately in the weeks and months to come, it's vital to take readings from the same place on each body part each time.

Chest: Place the tape measure around your chest so it runs across your nipples.
Waist: Place the tape measure around your waist so it runs straight across your tummy button.
Hips: Place the tape measure around your hips at the widest point.
Thigh: Place the tape measure around your leg at the highest part of your thigh, where it meets your groin.
Upper arm: Place the tape measure around your upper arm so it touches the highest part of your armpit.

WHAT IT ALL MEANS

Again, your waist measurement is the key one. A waist that measures 80cm (31½in) or over in women and 94cm (37in) or over in men puts you at increased risk of type-2 diabetes.

If your waist measures over 88cm (34.5in) for a woman and over 102cm (40in) for a man, you're in the high-risk zone for type-2 diabetes and heart disease.

The other four measurements will help you track your weight-loss progress – and provide a constant source of motivation.

MY MEASUREMENTS						
	Date	Chest	Waist	Hips	Thigh	Arm
Today						
After 1 week						
After 2 weeks						
After 3 weeks						
After 4 weeks						
After 5 weeks						
After 6 weeks						
After 7 weeks						
After 8 weeks						
After 9 weeks						
After 10 weeks						
After 3 months						
After 4 months						
After 5 months						
After 6 months						

TEST 3: WEIGHT AND BODY MASS INDEX (BMI)

WHAT YOU'LL NEED

- Pencil
- Tape measure
- Pen
- Scales (for consistency, always use the same set of scales)

WHY DO IT?

Your body mass index (BMI) expresses your weight in relation to your height and is used to work out whether you are overweight, underweight or just right for your height. It is sometimes criticized as not very accurate, because it doesn't directly take into account how much of your body weight is made up of fat and how much is made up of muscle. This means it can class very muscular but healthy people as overweight. However, for most of us, it's still a useful measurement, especially if you do it alongside the other tests that we recommend in this chapter.

WHAT TO DO

1. Stand against a wall in your bare feet and, placing the pencil on top of your head, use it to draw a line lightly on the wall. Now measure the distance from the floor to the mark with the tape measure to get your height, and note it down in the My Weight & BMI chart (see page 58).

2. Next, strip down to your underwear (or less, if you prefer), take a deep breath and hop on the scales. Now take another deep breath and open your eyes.

3. If you don't like what you see, don't despair. Simply tell yourself, 'This is the heaviest I'm ever going to be, so there's no need to panic. I'll never be this weight again.'

4. Now make a note on the My Weight & BMI chart of your weight (in either kilos or stones and pounds) and your weigh-in time and date, so that in future you can weigh yourself at more or less the same time of day.

5. Look at the Healthy Weight Range & BMI Table (pages 57 and 59) and calculate your BMI and healthy weight range – namely the area coloured green – and then fill in the rest of the chart overleaf.

6. Weigh yourself once a week and, for a really inspirational picture of your weight-loss progress, fill in the results on the graph on page 61. As your weight can fluctuate for a variety of reasons (such as how much you've just eaten or had to drink, whether you've just exercised, and so on), don't weigh yourself more than once a week, so your losses will have had time to accumulate.

HEALTHY WEIGHT RANGE & BMI TABLE

HEIGHT	BMI 15	16	17	18	19	20	21	22	23	24	25	26	27	28	29	30	31	32	33	34	35
1.47m 4ft 10in	32kg 5st	35kg 5st 7lb	37kg 5st 12lb	39kg 6st 2lb	41kg 6st 6lb	43kg 6st 11lb	45kg 7st 1lb	48kg 7st 8lb	50kg 7st 12lb	52kg 8st 3lb	54kg 8st 7lb	56kg 8st 12lb	58kg 9st 2lb	61kg 9st 9lb	63kg 9st 13lb	65kg 10st 3lb	67kg 10st 8lb	69kg 10st 12lb	71kg 11st 3lb	74kg 11st 9lb	76kg 12st
1.50m 4ft 11in	34kg 5st 5lb	36kg 5st 9lb	38kg 6st	40kg 6st 4lb	43kg 6st 11lb	45kg 7st 1lb	47kg 7st 6lb	49kg 7st 10lb	52kg 8st 3lb	54kg 8st 7lb	56kg 8st 12lb	59kg 9st 4lb	61kg 9st 9lb	63kg 9st 13lb	65kg 10st 3lb	68kg 10st 10lb	70kg 11st	72kg 11st 5lb	74kg 11st 9lb	76kg 12st	78kg 12st 4lb
1.52m 5ft	35kg 5st 7lb	37kg 5st 12lb	39kg 6st 2lb	42kg 6st 9lb	44kg 6st 13lb	46kg 7st 3lb	49kg 7st 10lb	51kg 8st	53kg 8st 5lb	55kg 8st 9lb	58kg 9st 2lb	60kg 9st 6lb	62kg 9st 11lb	65kg 10st 3lb	67kg 10st 8lb	69kg 10st 12lb	72kg 11st 5lb	74kg 11st 9lb	76kg 12st	79kg 12st 6lb	81kg 12st 11lb
1.55m 5ft 1in	36kg 5st 9lb	39kg 6st 2lb	41kg 6st 6lb	43kg 6st 11lb	46kg 7st 3lb	48kg 7st 8lb	50kg 7st 12lb	53kg 8st 5lb	55kg 8st 9lb	58kg 9st 2lb	60kg 9st 6lb	63kg 9st 13lb	65kg 10st 3lb	67kg 10st 8lb	69kg 10st 12lb	72kg 11st 5lb	74kg 11st 9lb	77kg 12st 2lb	79kg 12st 6lb	82kg 12st 13lb	84kg 13st 3lb
1.57m 5ft 2in	37kg 5st 12lb	40kg 6st 4lb	42kg 6st 9lb	44kg 6st 13lb	47kg 7st 6lb	49kg 7st 10lb	52kg 8st 3lb	54kg 8st 7lb	57kg 9st	59kg 9st 4lb	62kg 9st 11lb	64kg 10st 1lb	67kg 10st 8lb	69kg 10st 12lb	72kg 11st 5lb	74kg 11st 9lb	76kg 12st	79kg 12st 6lb	81kg 12st 11lb	84kg 13st 3lb	86kg 13st 8lb
1.6m 5ft 3in	39kg 6st 2lb	41kg 6st 6lb	44kg 6st 13lb	46kg 7st 3lb	49kg 7st 10lb	51kg 8st	54kg 8st 7lb	56kg 8st 12lb	59kg 9st 4lb	61kg 9st 9lb	64kg 10st 1lb	67kg 10st 8lb	69kg 10st 12lb	72kg 11st 5lb	74kg 11st 9lb	76kg 12st	79kg 12st 6lb	82kg 12st 13lb	84kg 13st 3lb	87kg 13st 10lb	90kg 14st 2lb
1.63m 5ft 4in	40kg 6st 4lb	42kg 6st 9lb	45kg 7st 1lb	48kg 7st 8lb	50kg 7st 12lb	53kg 8st 5lb	56kg 8st 12lb	58kg 9st 2lb	61kg 9st 9lb	64kg 10st 1lb	66kg 10st 6lb	69kg 10st 12lb	72kg 11st 5lb	74kg 11st 9lb	77kg 12st 2lb	80kg 12st 8lb	82kg 12st 13lb	85kg 13st 5lb	88kg 13st 12lb	90kg 14st 2lb	93kg 14st 9lb
1.65m 5ft 5in	41kg 6st 6lb	44kg 6st 13lb	46kg 7st 3lb	49kg 7st 10lb	52kg 8st 3lb	54kg 8st 7lb	57kg 9st	60kg 9st 6lb	63kg 9st 13lb	65kg 10st 3lb	68kg 10st 10lb	71kg 11st 3lb	73kg 11st 7lb	76kg 12st	79kg 12st 6lb	81kg 12st 11lb	84kg 13st 3lb	87kg 13st 10lb	90kg 14st 2lb	93kg 14st 9lb	95kg 14st 13lb
1.68m 5ft 6in	42kg 6st 9lb	45kg 7st 1lb	48kg 7st 8lb	51kg 8st	54kg 8st 7lb	56kg 8st 12lb	59kg 9st 4lb	62kg 9st 11lb	65kg 10st 3lb	68kg 10st 10lb	70kg 11st	73kg 11st 7lb	76kg 12st	79kg 12st 6lb	82kg 12st 13lb	84kg 13st 3lb	87kg 13st 10lb	90kg 14st 2lb	93kg 14st 9lb	96kg 15st 2lb	99kg 15st 8lb

Healthy weight range

MY WEIGHT & BMI

	My height
	My healthy weight range

	Date/ weigh-in time	Weight	Weight loss	BMI	Dress/ waist size
Today					
After 1 week					
After 2 weeks					
After 3 weeks					
After 4 weeks					
After 5 weeks					
After 6 weeks					
After 7 weeks					
After 8 weeks					
After 9 weeks					
After 10 weeks					
After 3 months					
After 4 months					
After 5 months					
After 6 months					

HEALTHY WEIGHT RANGE & BMI TABLE

HEIGHT (BMI)	15	16	17	18	19	20	21	22	23	24	25	26	27	28	29	30	31	32	33	34	35
1.7m / 5ft 7in	44kg 6st 13lb	46kg 7st 3lb	49kg 7st 10lb	52kg 8st 3lb	55kg 8st 9lb	58kg 9st 2lb	61kg 9st 9lb	63kg 9st 13lb	67kg 10st 8lb	69kg 10st 12lb	72kg 11st 5lb	75kg 11st 11lb	78kg 12st 4lb	81kg 12st 11lb	84kg 13st 3lb	87kg 13st 10lb	90kg 14st 2lb	93kg 14st 9lb	96kg 15st 2lb	98kg 15st 6lb	101kg 15st 13lb
1.73m / 5ft 8in	45kg 7st 1lb	48kg 7st 8lb	51kg 8st	54kg 8st 7lb	57kg 9st	60kg 9st 6lb	63kg 9st 13lb	66kg 10st 6lb	69kg 10st 12lb	72kg 11st 5lb	75kg 11st 11lb	78kg 12st 4lb	81kg 12st 11lb	84kg 13st 3lb	87kg 13st 10lb	90kg 14st 2lb	93kg 14st 9lb	96kg 15st 2lb	99kg 15st 8lb	102kg 16st 1lb	105kg 16st 8lb
1.75m / 5ft 9in	46kg 7st 3lb	49kg 7st 10lb	52kg 8st 3lb	55kg 8st 9lb	58kg 9st 2lb	61kg 9st 9lb	64kg 10st 1lb	68kg 10st 10lb	71kg 11st 3lb	74kg 11st 9lb	76kg 12st	80kg 12st 8lb	83kg 13st 1lb	86kg 13st 8lb	89kg 14st	92kg 14st 7lb	95kg 14st 13lb	98kg 15st 6lb	101kg 15st 13lb	104kg 16st 5lb	107kg 16st 12lb
1.78m / 5ft 10in	48kg 7st 8lb	51kg 8st	54kg 8st 7lb	57kg 9st	60kg 9st 6lb	63kg 9st 13lb	67kg 10st 8lb	70kg 11st	73kg 11st 7lb	76kg 12st	79kg 12st 6lb	82kg 12st 13lb	86kg 13st 8lb	89kg 14st	92kg 14st 7lb	95kg 14st 13lb	98kg 15st 6lb	101kg 15st 13lb	105kg 16st 8lb	108kg 17st	111kg 17st 7lb
1.8m / 5ft 11in	49kg 7st 10lb	52kg 8st 3lb	55kg 8st 9lb	58kg 9st 2lb	62kg 9st 11lb	65kg 10st 3lb	68kg 10st 10lb	72kg 11st 5lb	75kg 11st 11lb	78kg 12st 4lb	81kg 12st 11lb	84kg 13st 3lb	87kg 13st 10lb	91kg 14st 5lb	94kg 14st 11lb	98kg 15st 6lb	101kg 15st 13lb	104kg 16st 5lb	107kg 16st 12lb	110kg 17st 5lb	113kg 17st 11lb
1.83m / 6ft	50kg 7st 12lb	54kg 8st 7lb	57kg 9st	60kg 9st 6lb	63kg 9st 13lb	67kg 10st 8lb	70kg 11st	73kg 11st 7lb	77kg 12st 2lb	80kg 12st 8lb	83kg 13st	87kg 13st 10lb	90kg 14st 2lb	94kg 14st 11lb	97kg 15st 4lb	100kg 15st 10lb	104kg 16st 5lb	107kg 16st 12lb	111kg 17st 7lb	114kg 17st 13lb	117kg 18st 6lb
1.85m / 6ft 1in	51kg 8st	55kg 8st 9lb	59kg 9st 4lb	62kg 9st 11lb	65kg 10st 3lb	69kg 10st 12lb	72kg 11st 5lb	76kg 12st	79kg 12st 6lb	82kg 12st 13lb	86kg 13st 8lb	89kg 14st	93kg 14st 9lb	96kg 15st 2lb	100kg 15st 10lb	103kg 16st 3lb	106kg 16st 10lb	110kg 17st 5lb	113kg 17st 11lb	117kg 18st 6lb	120kg 18st 13lb
1.88m / 6ft 2in	53kg 8st 5lb	57kg 9st	60kg 9st 6lb	64kg 10st 1lb	67kg 10st 8lb	71kg 11st 3lb	74kg 11st 9lb	78kg 12st 4lb	81kg 12st 11lb	84kg 13st 3lb	88kg 13st 12lb	92kg 14st 7lb	95kg 14st 13lb	99kg 15st 8lb	103kg 16st 3lb	106kg 16st 10lb	110kg 17st 5lb	113kg 17st 11lb	117kg 18st 6lb	120kg 18st 13lb	124kg 19st 7lb
1.9m / 6ft 3in	54kg 8st 7lb	58kg 9st 2lb	62kg 9st 11lb	65kg 10st 3lb	69kg 10st 12lb	73kg 11st 7lb	76kg 12st	80kg 12st 8lb	83kg 13st 1lb	87kg 13st 10lb	91kg 14st 5lb	94kg 14st 11lb	98kg 15st 6lb	101kg 15st 13lb	105kg 16st 8lb	109kg 17st 2lb	112kg 17st 9lb	116kg 18st 4lb	120kg 18st 13lb	123kg 19st 6lb	126kg 19st 12lb
1.93m / 6ft 4in	56kg 8st 12lb	60kg 9st 6lb	63kg 9st 13lb	67kg 10st 8lb	71kg 11st 3lb	74kg 11st 9lb	78kg 12st 4lb	82kg 12st 13lb	86kg 13st 8lb	89kg 14st	93kg 14st 9lb	97kg 15st 4lb	101kg 15st 13lb	104kg 16st 5lb	107kg 16st 12lb	112kg 17st 9lb	116kg 18st 4lb	119kg 18st 10lb	123kg 19st 6lb	127kg 20st	130kg 20st 6lb

Healthy weight range (BMI 19–24)

Adapted from a BMI chart supplied courtesy of Weight Watchers (www.weightwatchers.co.uk)

TEST 4: BODY-FAT PERCENTAGE

WHAT YOU'LL NEED
- Pen
- Scales with a body-fat monitor function (for consistency, always use the same ones)

OR

- Gym membership or access to a personal trainer

This test measures the percentage of fat in your body. It's the only one of the four tests that requires specialist equipment (or a personal trainer or gym membership), which can be expensive, so don't worry if you can't manage to do it. However, remember that being able to see that your body fat is burning off and your muscle tissue is increasing is highly motivating and will give you a more accurate picture of your health.

WHY DO IT?
Simply measuring your weight alone isn't a clear indicator of good health because ordinary scales aren't psychic – they can't tell the difference between weight that comes from fat and weight that comes from lean body tissue (muscles, bones, organs and blood). This means it's possible for your weight to be in the ideal range yet your body-fat level to be on the high side. Why is it important to be aware of how much body fat you have? Well, if your level is excessively high, you're at risk of getting some very nasty diseases such as heart disease, arthritis, type-2 diabetes and some types of cancer, and the risk soars as your body-fat level increases. If your

body fat is excessively low, this can lead to increased risk of osteoporosis, a decrease in fertility and even amenorrhoea, a condition in which women cease to have periods.

Something else to bear in mind is that 450g (1lb) of fat tissue burns only two calories in 24 hours, whereas 450g (1lb) of muscle burns about 35 calories, so the more muscle you have, the more calories you'll burn. Adding just a little muscle makes a big difference to the number of calories you use a day. A kilo (2lb) of muscle burns an extra 70 calories a day – that's 2,100 calories per month, equivalent to losing 225g (more than half a pound) of fat. And that's without changing your diet!

Monitoring your body fat is really helpful if you're trying to lose weight and don't seem to be getting anywhere (been there, done that?) because it will prove to you that your workout plan is actually working. It'll show you that you're replacing fat with muscle, which, because it's heavier than fat, can make you despair at having gained weight.

HOW IS IT DONE?
Body fat can be measured in a variety of ways. One method involves using a body-fat monitor, which works on the principle of bioelectrical impedance analysis (BIA). It sounds scary, but what this means is that a very low, safe, painless electrical signal is passed through your body (however, it shouldn't be used by pregnant women or those with pacemakers). This signal

passes through the fluids in lean tissue but has difficulty getting through fat tissue. The body-fat monitor measures this difficulty (hence the term bio-electrical impedance) and then uses the additional information you've given it, such as your sex and height, to calculate your body-fat percentage. The good news is that body-fat monitors aren't available solely to gym-goers and athletes – you can use one in the privacy of your own home. Tanita makes the best-known brand of monitor, which handily doubles up as conventional scales (29% of Japanese people own one!). Another reputable but less well-known brand is Salter. (For stockists, visit www.tanita.com and www.salterhousewares.com.)

WHAT TO DO

If you have scales that double as a body-fat monitor, programme them according to the instructions and take your reading. Always do the test at the same time of day so you're comparing like with like. The best time to do this test is in the early evening, before a meal, when you're more likely to be fully hydrated. Follow the manufacturer's instructions to the letter, as things such as not going to the loo before the test or when you last ate or drank can distort your results. This is because these things can raise or lower the amount of water in your body, which affects the amount of resistance it'll put up to the electrical signal. Alternatively, ask an instructor at your gym (or a personal trainer) to do the test for you.

MY BODY-FAT PERCENTAGE		
	Date / time	Body-fat percentage
Today		
After 1 week		
After 2 weeks		
After 3 weeks		
After 4 weeks		
After 5 weeks		
After 6 weeks		
After 7 weeks		
After 8 weeks		
After 9 weeks		
After 10 weeks		
After 3 months		
After 4 months		
After 5 months		
After 6 months		

WHAT IT ALL MEANS

▶▶

This chart will give you an indication of the healthy ranges to aim for:

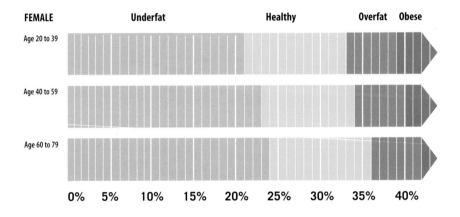

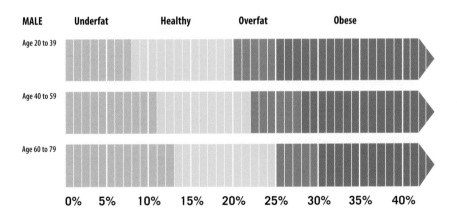

National Institutes of Health/World Health Organisation BMI guidelines, as reported by Gallagher at the New York Obesity Research Center, based on data from the *American Journal of Clinical Nutrition* 2000; 72: 694-701. Data used with permission of the *American Journal of Clinical Nutrition* © Am J Clin Nutr American Society For Clinical Nutrition

AND FINALLY ...

▶▶

Once you've done all the tests, fill in your scores on the 'How I Measure Up Today' chart (below), then after six months' worth of exercise and tests, fill in the 'How I Measure Up In Six Months Time' chart (below) to see exactly how much progress you've made. We guarantee you'll be amazed!

HOW I MEASURE UP TODAY	
Today's date	
Dress/ clothing size	
Weight	
BMI	
Body-fat percentage	
Resting heart rate	
Body measurements	
Chest	
Waist	
Hips	
Thigh	
Arm	

HOW I MEASURE UP IN SIX MONTHS' TIME	
Today's date	
Dress/ clothing size	
Weight	
BMI	
Body-fat percentage	
Resting heart rate	
Body measurements	
Chest	
Waist	
Hips	
Thigh	
Arm	

HERE'S THE MOMENT YOU'VE BEEN
WAITING FOR – YOU'RE ABOUT TO
MEET YOUR PERFECT RUNNING PLAN
AND TAKE YOUR FIRST STEPS
TOWARDS A NEW, IMPROVED YOU ...

6. GET GOING

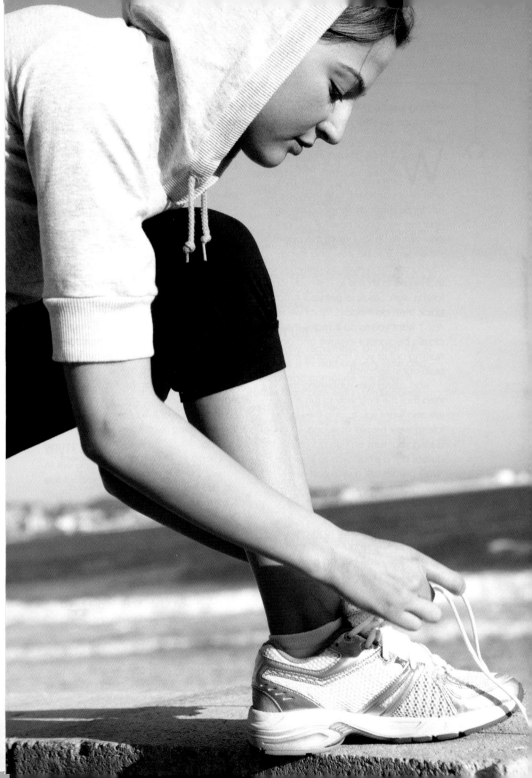

YOUR FILL-IT-IN 60-SECOND-SECRET PLAN
(complete with Mood-O-Meter)

USE OUR UNIQUE MOOD-O-METER TO MEASURE YOUR MOOD BEFORE, DURING AND AFTER
EVERY RUN AND YOU'LL SOON REALIZE THAT EVEN ON THOSE DAYS WHEN RUNNING FEELS LIKE
THE VERY LAST THING YOU WANT TO DO, YOU'LL ABSOLUTELY ALWAYS FEEL LIKE A MILLION
DOLLARS AFTERWARDS. READ ON TO DISCOVER WHAT THE SYMBOLS (BELOW) REALLY MEAN ...

HOW YOU FELT ... BEFORE YOUR RUN

HELLISH
Wild horses had to drag me out of the door. I did not want to run today.

INDIFFERENT
I went out because I was scheduled to, not because I wanted to.

UP AND DOWN
I was in two minds whether to go running or not.

GOOD
I had no problem getting going today – I felt fit and positive.

EUPHORIC
I was itching to go out for a run – nothing could hold me back.

HOW YOU FELT ... DURING YOUR RUN

HELLISH
That was simply awful! I loathed every second. My breath came in ragged gasps and I had logs for legs.

INDIFFERENT
That was the equivalent of a school dinner – dull and uneventful.

UP AND DOWN
There were bad bits, but good bits, too. As soon as I got going, I felt better.

GOOD
I enjoyed my run – my legs felt strong and I felt in control the whole time.

EUPHORIC
Running? I was flying! Hill? What hill? I could have gone on for ever – and then some.

HOW YOU FELT ... AFTER YOUR RUN

HELLISH
Eugh! I really hated that and felt terrible afterwards.

INDIFFERENT
Errrr, that was a bit grim. But it was bearable ... I guess.

UP AND DOWN
Hmmm, I loved and hated it in equal measure.

GOOD
I felt great – relaxed, invigorated and extremely proud of myself.

EUPHORIC
Wow! I felt elated and couldn't wait to go and do it all over again.

WEEK ONE

'The miracle isn't that I finished – the miracle is that I had the courage to start'

John Bingham, motivational expert

MONDAY Run 60 secs, walk 3 mins. Repeat 3 more times   (Total: 16 mins)
Time of day you're planning to run: _____   Mood before: ☹😐😑🙂😄
Mood during: ☹😐😑🙂😄
Daily Reward _____   Mood after: ☹😐😑🙂😄

TUESDAY Rest

WEDNESDAY Run 60 secs, walk 3 mins. Repeat 3 more times   (Total: 16 mins)
Time of day you're planning to run: _____   Mood before: ☹😐😑🙂😄
Mood during: ☹😐😑🙂😄
Daily Reward _____   Mood after: ☹😐😑🙂😄

THURSDAY Rest

FRIDAY Run 60 secs, walk 3 mins. Repeat 3 more times   (Total: 16 mins)
Time of day you're planning to run: _____   Mood before: ☹😐😑🙂😄
Mood during: ☹😐😑🙂😄
Daily Reward _____   Mood after: ☹😐😑🙂😄

SATURDAY Rest

SUNDAY 30-minute brisk walk
Time of day you're planning to run: _____   Mood before: ☹😐😑🙂😄
Mood during: ☹😐😑🙂😄
Weekly Treat _____   Mood after: ☹😐😑🙂😄

You may be feeling ... weak and wobbly. You may feel like Bambi on ice (both during and after your session!), and your bottom may feel as if it's jiggling around like jelly on a plate, but don't let this put you off. It's only a temporary phase as running is one of the fastest ways on the planet to get fit and firm up. Even really experienced runners feel bad after a long lay-off. It really doesn't matter what you look or feel like right now the important thing, as the quote above says, is that you've had the courage to start.

'If you want to become the best runner you can be, start now'

Priscilla Welch, marathon runner

MONDAY Run 60 secs, walk 2 mins. Repeat 5 more times (Total: 18 mins)
Time of day you're planning to run: _____ Mood before: ☹️😐😕😊😄
  Mood during: ☹️😐😕😊😄
Daily Reward _____ Mood after: ☹️😐😕😊😄

TUESDAY Rest

WEDNESDAY Run 60 secs, walk 2 mins. Repeat 5 more times (Total: 18 mins)
Time of day you're planning to run: _____ Mood before: ☹️😐😕😊😄
  Mood during: ☹️😐😕😊😄
Daily Reward _____ Mood after: ☹️😐😕😊😄

THURSDAY Rest

FRIDAY Run 60 secs, walk 3 mins. Repeat 3 more times (Total: 16 mins)
Time of day you're planning to run: _____ Mood before: ☹️😐😕😊😄
  Mood during: ☹️😐😕😊😄
Daily Reward _____ Mood after: ☹️😐😕😊😄

SATURDAY Rest

SUNDAY 30-minute brisk walk
Time of day you're planning to run: _____ Mood before: ☹️😐😕😊😄
  Mood during: ☹️😐😕😊😄
Weekly Treat _____ Mood after: ☹️😐😕😊😄

You may be feeling ... puffed out. But this is perfectly normal – you'll need to breathe a bit faster because your body needs more oxygen to fuel its efforts. (As you get fitter, you'll definitely feel less breathless.) However, you shouldn't be gasping for breath – if you're practically hyperventilating, just slow down and do what you can. A simple way to make sure you're not overdoing it is to take the Talk Test. If you can talk, you're running at the right pace, but if you can sing, you're not making enough effort.

WEEK THREE

'Remember, a step forward, no matter how small, is a step in the right direction'

Kara Goucher, long-distance runner

MONDAY 60 secs, walk 2 mins. Repeat 6 more times   (Total: 21 mins)
Time of day you're planning to run: _____   Mood before: ☹️😐😏🙂😄
                                                          Mood during: ☹️😐😏🙂😄
Daily Reward _____   Mood after: ☹️😐😏🙂😄

TUESDAY Rest

WEDNESDAY 60 secs, walk 2 mins. Repeat 6 more times   (Total: 21 mins)
Time of day you're planning to run: _____   Mood before: ☹️😐😏🙂😄
                                                          Mood during: ☹️😐😏🙂😄
Daily Reward _____   Mood after: ☹️😐😏🙂😄

THURSDAY Rest

FRIDAY 60 secs, walk 2 mins. Repeat 6 more times   (Total: 21 mins)
Time of day you're planning to run: _____   Mood before: ☹️😐😏🙂😄
                                                          Mood during: ☹️😐😏🙂😄
Daily Reward _____   Mood after: ☹️😐😏🙂😄

SATURDAY Rest

SUNDAY 30-minute brisk walk
Time of day you're planning to run: _____   Mood before: ☹️😐😏🙂😄
                                                          Mood during: ☹️😐😏🙂😄
Weekly Treat _____   Mood after: ☹️😐😏🙂😄

You may be feeling ... stiff and sore. Muscles that you never knew you had will come kicking and screaming to the surface and demand your attention. Make sure you help your body to adapt by always stretching properly after every run (see tip 54 in Chapter 7), and try soaking in a warm bath to get rid of aches and pains. And if you have some spare cash, treat yourself to a massage to help soothe sore muscles and get you feeling blissfully relaxed.

WEEK FOUR

'Running is the greatest metaphor for life, because you get out of it what you put into it'

Oprah Winfrey, US media mogul

MONDAY Run 60 secs, walk 2 mins. Repeat 7 more times   (Total: 24 mins)
Time of day you're planning to run:_____   Mood before: 😟😐😑🙂😄
Mood during: 😟😐😑🙂😄
Daily Reward _____   Mood after: 😟😐😑🙂😄

TUESDAY Rest

WEDNESDAY Run 60 secs, walk 2 mins. Repeat 7 more times   (Total: 24 mins)
Time of day you're planning to run: _____   Mood before: 😟😐😑🙂😄
Mood during: 😟😐😑🙂😄
Daily Reward _____   Mood after: 😟😐😑🙂😄

THURSDAY Rest

FRIDAY Run 60 secs, walk 2 mins. Repeat 7 more times   (Total: 24 mins)
Time of day you're planning to run:_____   Mood before: 😟😐😑🙂😄
Mood during: 😟😐😑🙂😄
Daily Reward _____   Mood after: 😟😐😑🙂😄

SATURDAY Rest

SUNDAY 35-minute brisk walk
Time of day you're planning to run:_____   Mood before: 😟😐😑🙂😄
Mood during: 😟😐😑🙂😄
Weekly Treat _____   Mood after: 😟😐😑🙂😄

You may be feeling ... unsure if you're really doing it right, if it's ever going to work – or even if you want to continue doing it at all. Don't worry, everyone has beginner's doubts. Stick at it – your confidence, like your fitness, will grow every time you finish a session until running starts feeling like the most natural thing in the world.

WEEK FIVE

'Whether you believe you can or believe you can't, you're probably right'

Henry Ford, industrialist

MONDAY 60 secs, walk 2 mins. Repeat 8 more times
Time of day you're planning to run:_____

Daily Reward _____

(Total: 27 mins)
Mood before: ☹️😕😐🙂😄
Mood during: ☹️😕😐🙂😄
Mood after: ☹️😕😐🙂😄

TUESDAY Rest

WEDNESDAY Swap in a different kind of exercise session here – do anything from brisk walking, swimming or cycling to weights or an aerobics class. Aim for a 30-minute gentle workout – doing either just one activity or a mix of two 15-minute or three 10-minute workouts adding up to 30 minutes
Time of day you're planning to run: _____

Daily Reward _____

Mood before: ☹️😕😐🙂😄
Mood during: ☹️😕😐🙂😄
Mood after: ☹️😕😐🙂😄

THURSDAY Rest

FRIDAY 60 secs, walk 2 mins. Repeat 8 more times
Time of day you're planning to run:_____

Daily Reward _____

(Total: 27 mins)
Mood before: ☹️😕😐🙂😄
Mood during: ☹️😕😐🙂😄
Mood after: ☹️😕😐🙂😄

SATURDAY Rest

SUNDAY 60 secs, walk 2 mins. Repeat 8 more times
Time of day you're planning to run:_____

Weekly Treat _____

(Total: 27 mins)
Mood before: ☹️😕😐🙂😄
Mood during: ☹️😕😐🙂😄
Mood after: ☹️😕😐🙂😄

You may be feeling ... like giving up. Don't! You've come halfway and it'll all get easier from now on. When you're feeling weak-willed, think back to how much effort you've made and what a shame it would be to waste it. Think about how far you've already come – admit it, just a few weeks ago the thought of exercising for 30 minutes was enough to turn your stomach!

WEEK SIX

'No one can say, "You must not run faster than this …" The human spirit is indomitable'

Sir Roger Bannister, athlete

MONDAY Run 2 mins, walk 2 mins. Repeat 6 more times   (Total: 28 mins)
Time of day you're planning to run: _____   Mood before: ☹☹☺☺☺
Mood during: ☹☹☺☺☺
Daily Reward _____   Mood after: ☹☹☺☺☺

TUESDAY Rest

WEDNESDAY Free session – 30 minutes' brisk walking/dancing/cycling/
swimming/weights – whatever you like!
Time of day you're planning to run: _____   Mood before: ☹☹☺☺☺
Mood during: ☹☹☺☺☺
Daily Reward _____   Mood after: ☹☹☺☺☺

THURSDAY Rest

FRIDAY Run 2 mins, walk 2 mins. Repeat 6 more times   (Total: 28 mins)
Time of day you're planning to run: _____   Mood before: ☹☹☺☺☺
Mood during: ☹☹☺☺☺
Daily Reward _____   Mood after: ☹☹☺☺☺

SATURDAY Rest

SUNDAY Run 2 mins, walk 2 mins. Repeat 6 more times   (Total: 28 mins)
Time of day you're planning to run: _____   Mood before: ☹☹☺☺☺
Mood during: ☹☹☺☺☺
Weekly Treat _____   Mood after: ☹☹☺☺☺

You may be feeling ... sweaty, especially as you're now having to get used to running for 2 minutes at a stretch. But don't be grossed out by your own sweat – see it rather as a badge of courage, something you've earned. Remember that you can lose up to 500ml/1 pint of sweat per 30-minute workout, so drink plenty of water before, during and after your sessions. Experts recommend that you drink between half a teacup to a teacup every ten to 20 minutes when you're exercising.

WEEK SEVEN

'My philosophy on running is, I don't dwell on it, I do it'

Joan Benoit Samuelson, marathon runner

MONDAY Run 2 mins, walk 2 mins. Repeat 7 more times   (Total: 32 mins)

Time of day you're planning to run: _____

Mood before: ☹😐😑🙂😄
Mood during: ☹😐😑🙂😄

Daily Reward _____

Mood after: ☹😐😑🙂😄

TUESDAY Rest

WEDNESDAY Free session – 30 minutes to do a fun activity!

Time of day you're planning to run: _____

Mood before: ☹😐😑🙂😄
Mood during: ☹😐😑🙂😄

Daily Reward _____

Mood after: ☹😐😑🙂😄

THURSDAY Rest

FRIDAY Run 2 mins, walk 2 mins. Repeat 7 more times   (Total: 32 mins)

Time of day you're planning to run:_____

Mood before: ☹😐😑🙂😄
Mood during: ☹😐😑🙂😄

Daily Reward _____

Mood after: ☹😐😑🙂😄

SATURDAY Rest

SUNDAY Run 2 mins, walk 2 mins. Repeat 7 more times   (Total: 32 mins)

Time of day you're planning to run: _____

Mood before: ☹😐😑🙂😄
Mood during: ☹😐😑🙂😄

Weekly Treat _____

Mood after: ☹😐😑🙂😄

You may be feeling ... guilty for missing a session. Don't give yourself a hard time about it – that will simply make you feel bad and you'll be less likely to want to stick with the programme. Don't dwell on past mistakes – run away from them! There's nothing like simply getting out and running the next day to ease your conscience.

WEEK EIGHT

'He who is not courageous enough to take risks will accomplish nothing in life'

Muhammad Ali, boxer

MONDAY Run 3 mins, walk 2 mins. Repeat 6 more times
Time of day you're planning to run: _____

Daily Reward _____

(Total: 35 mins)
Mood before: ☹😐😑😊😄
Mood during: ☹😐😑😊😄
Mood after: ☹😐😑😊😄

TUESDAY Rest

WEDNESDAY Try to increase your free session to 40 minutes – have fun!
Time of day you're planning to run: _____

Daily Reward _____

Mood before: ☹😐😑😊😄
Mood during: ☹😐😑😊😄
Mood after: ☹😐😑😊😄

THURSDAY Rest

FRIDAY Run 3 mins, walk 2 mins. Repeat 6 more times
Time of day you're planning to run: _____

Daily Reward _____

(Total: 35 mins)
Mood before: ☹😐😑😊😄
Mood during: ☹😐😑😊😄
Mood after: ☹😐😑😊😄

SATURDAY Rest

SUNDAY Run 3 mins, walk 2 mins. Repeat 6 more times
Time of day you're planning to run: _____

Weekly Treat _____

(Total: 35 mins)
Mood before: ☹😐😑😊😄
Mood during: ☹😐😑😊😄
Mood after: ☹😐😑😊😄

You may be feeling ... impatient, that the programme's holding you back rather than helping you move forward – but we promise it's not. What it's doing is making sure your body is ready to take running to another level, and that you aren't injured. We guarantee you'll get to run further once your body's ready, and that you'll be able to tackle races and even marathons (if you want a preview, check out Chapter 8). Bear with us, because good things come to those who wait. You're well on your way to acquiring the exercise habit – which is even more important than simply getting fit.

WEEK NINE

'The woods are lovely dark and deep, but I have … miles to go before I sleep'

Robert Frost, poet

MONDAY Run 3 mins, walk 2 mins. Repeat 6 more times (Total: 35 mins)
Time of day you're planning to run: _____   Mood before: ☹😐😑🙂😄
Mood during: ☹😐😑🙂😄
Daily Reward _____   Mood after: ☹😐😑🙂😄

TUESDAY Rest

WEDNESDAY Free session – 40 minutes of any activity you choose
Time of day you're planning to run: _____   Mood before: ☹😐😑🙂😄
Mood during: ☹😐😑🙂😄
Daily Reward _____   Mood after: ☹😐😑🙂😄

THURSDAY Rest

FRIDAY Run 3 mins, walk 60 secs. Repeat 8 more times (Total: 36 mins)
Time of day you're planning to run: _____   Mood before: ☹😐😑🙂😄
Mood during: ☹😐😑🙂😄
Daily Reward _____   Mood after: ☹😐😑🙂😄

SATURDAY Rest

SUNDAY Run 3 mins, walk 60 secs. Repeat 8 more times (Total: 36 mins)
Time of day you're planning to run: _____   Mood before: ☹😐😑🙂😄
Mood during: ☹😐😑🙂😄
Weekly Treat _____   Mood after: ☹😐😑🙂😄

You may be feeling … slimmer. If weight loss was one of your goals, this should please you no end – and make you even more enthusiastic to finish the programme. Running is a fabulously efficient fat burner so by now you're likely to start seeing and feeling the difference. Book an appointment with your bank manager today – you're going to need an overdraft to finance your new wardrobe of sized-down clothes!

WEEK TEN

'I celebrate myself'

Walt Whitman, poet

MONDAY Run 3 mins, walk 60 secs. Repeat 8 more times   (Total: 36 mins)
Time of day you're planning to run: _____   Mood before: ☹️😐😑🙂😄
   Mood during: ☹️😐😑🙂😄
Daily Reward _____   Mood after: ☹️😐😑🙂😄

TUESDAY Rest

WEDNESDAY Free session – 40 minutes to do whatever exercise you like!
Time of day you're planning to run: _____   Mood before: ☹️😐😑🙂😄
   Mood during: ☹️😐😑🙂😄
Daily Reward _____   Mood after: ☹️😐😑🙂😄

THURSDAY Rest

FRIDAY Run 3 mins, walk 60 secs. Repeat 8 more times   (Total: 36 mins)
Time of day you're planning to run: _____   Mood before: ☹️😐😑🙂😄
   Mood during: ☹️😐😑🙂�😄
Daily Reward _____   Mood after: ☹️😐😑🙂😄

SATURDAY Rest

SUNDAY Run 3 mins, walk 60 secs. Repeat 9 more times   (Total: 40 mins)
Time of day you're planning to run: _____   Mood before: ☹️😐😑🙂😄
   Mood during: ☹️😐😑🙂😄
Ultimate Indulgence!_____   Mood after: ☹️😐😑🙂😄

You may be feeling ... elated. And so you should! WELL DONE! You've reached your first goal and can now walk and run for up to 40 minutes and should easily be able to complete a 5K (3-mile) race. Why not try a Race For Life (visit www.raceforlife.org); go along to your nearest Parkrun on a Saturday morning for a free, weekly, 5K timed run (visit www.parkrun.org.uk); or join a RunEngland group (visit www.runengland.info)? Isn't it amazing what a difference 60 seconds can make?

'WE TRIED IT!'

THESE PEOPLE HAVE PUT THE 60-SECOND-SECRET PLAN THROUGH ITS PACES – HERE'S HOW THEY FOUND IT ...

'I've never been very good at PE or sticking to an exercise routine, so I was surprised to find myself really enjoying the plan. What I like the best is that it's easy to fit into your day. It never felt hard to run for 60 seconds and using the Mood-O-Meter proved to me just how much I was enjoying the sessions. Although on a few days I circled the Indifferent and Up And Down faces before my session, I always found myself circling the Good and Euphoric faces to sum up how great I felt while I was running along. For my rewards, I'd have a nice long soak in the bath before getting dressed up to go out for the night, or I'd watch *The Big Bang Theory*.'
Talia Wood, 21, journalism student, London

'I always loved the idea of being able to run long distances but always thought I couldn't do it, even though I'd tried a few times. Then I bought the first version of *Running Made Easy* and followed the plan to get to 5K and did it, I was so chuffed with myself. What I didn't realize was that after the first 10 minutes or so of running your body settles into it, breathing becomes easier and you can just keep going – I wish someone had told me that years ago and maybe I wouldn't have given up after a few minutes when I'd tried in the past.'
Paula Hale, 45, freelance gardener, Merseyside

'Before I started The 60-Second-Secret Plan, I hadn't run for three years because of a knee injury. When I first saw the programme, I thought, "I'm an international water-polo player, it's way too easy," but then I remembered that although I was fit, I'd barely run a step in three years. At times, I was tempted to run rather than walk but I kept reminding myself to take it slowly. I felt thrilled after each and every session as I went farther every time and, joy of joys, remained pain-free. Having finished the programme, I'm now able to run 5K (3 miles) effortlessly and it's even made a difference to my water-polo as my legs are stronger.'
Guy Mottram, 37, legal adviser, Johannesburg, South Africa

'I tried running for the first time aged 55 but, after only a few weeks, I had to give up because of a problem with my Achilles tendon. I then followed the ten-week plan in *Running Made Easy* and I realized that I had been trying to improve too quickly. The plan seemed too easy, but if you stick with it you really are training your body to run injury free. Legitimizing walk breaks made all the difference and I now run regularly injury free.'
Evelyn Leslie, 57, teacher, Cheshire

'HOW I GOT STARTED'

STILL FEELING NERVOUS ABOUT MAKING YOUR RUNNING DEBUT? REMEMBER, EVERYONE WAS A BEGINNER ONCE. TAKE A LOOK AT HOW THESE RUNNERS GOT STARTED, AND THEN JUST DO IT!

'I did my first run in Brighton when I was 20. I went downhill towards the sea, fast, in the wrong shoes, and ended up with sore shins. One good pair of shoes and mended shins later, I ran on the flat promenade, slowly, for what seemed like hours. Five minutes after I'd started, I arrived home. **My face was a terrifying colour, but I knew I was on to something.** And I was right. Fifteen years later, I'm still running. I've never run a race, nor do I aim to beat my times or run when I don't feel like it – because to me, running should be all about pleasure.'
Allie Packer, 35, journalist, London

'When I turned 30, I thought the world had come to an end. **In a desperate attempt to ward off old age, I started running.** Clad in a white-and-brown mini-dress and tackies (tennis shoes), I became an odd but familiar sight in my neighbourhood at a time when running wasn't as popular among ordinary women as it is today. Thirty-three years later, I completed the New York City Marathon with my two daughters. My running gear has changed but that is about all.'
Leone Jackson, 64, tour guide, Pretoria, South Africa

'A few years ago I was 136.5kg (21st 7lb) and ridiculously unhealthy. As well as changing what I was eating and making healthier choices, I started parking further away from where I worked and walking in, increasing the distance as I got lighter and quicker. Walking soon became my 'thing' but it wasn't long before I felt I needed to push myself harder. **I started jogging, and eventually running, and before long I found I really enjoyed running in organized events.** I've now lost over 44.5kg (7st) and I love running so much that I've completed a half-marathon and entered two more, and have signed up for the Beachy Head Marathon in October. Entering events keeps me focused and makes me really keen to train, regardless of the conditions!'
Colin Evans, 44, team leader, Kent

'I started running because **I was determined to lose weight.** Initially, I wobbled everywhere but now the extra 19kg (3st) I had put on has vanished and I'm trim and the happiest I've ever been. I know I'll never be Paula Radcliffe, but with running in my life, I'll always be a better version of me.'
Kat Arney, 27, scientist, London

'It was all the builders' fault! They came at 7.30am – in the middle of winter, too. I faced a stark choice – to sit in the kitchen huddled over a cup of tea or go for a walk. The walk won. After a few days, this seemed too slow and cold, so a faster shuffle was called for. **Before I knew it, I was running (slowly),** round a 3K (2 mile) circuit. By the time the builders left, I was hooked. Four marathons later, I still ask myself why I do it. My family think I'm mad to lay myself open to blisters, black toenails and 42.2K (26.2 miles) of slog. But I guess the buzz I get from joining like-minded mad people in hurling ourselves down a road has to be experienced to be appreciated.'
Rosemary Beach, 63, tour guide, Oxford

'In late December 2012 my father had a heart attack. He pulled through but **it made me realize that I couldn't carry on the way I was.** I was an occasional gym-goer and could be seen even less often on the rugby pitch at prop forward. I was 178cm (5ft 10in), 33 years old and weighed nearly 121kg (19st). In January 2013, I decided to enter the Big Fun Run in Milton Keynes and got a few mates to sign up with me. I tried spending more time at the gym but I hated the overcrowded changing rooms and the unavailable equipment. So in April I decided to hit the road, got an app for my phone and tracked my runs. A really good friend asked me to do a local 5K (3 mile) fun run with him in May and I never looked back. Running has and is changing my life. I am now in touch with old friends mainly through running and am now a more sensible, but still a long-way-to-go, 95kg (15st). Last year I managed my first half-marathon and clocked in at 1:52, which according to Run Britain is in the top 42% of UK times.'
Kelvin Chadwick, 34, warehouseman, Bedfordshire

'Needing to do exercise of some sort, I joined a group of eight local long-distance runners and for 20 years **we ran together, doing runs that were filled with wonderful camaraderie, banter and reminiscences.** Even when some of us got too old to run, we continued to meet for dinner every two months. Now there are only two of us left but, along with our wives and two of the widows, we still meet as regularly and remember the others who have crossed the finish line before us. There's no doubt that my running years were a highlight of my life. The memories of all the hours together on the road with my friends, the happy nonsense that was talked and the experiences we shared, are still, and always will be, with me.'
David Pistorius, 74, lawyer, Durban, South Africa

'HOW I FIND THE TIME TO RUN'

ALWAYS GOT A MILLION AND ONE THINGS COMPETING FOR YOUR TIME EVERY DAY? HERE, RUNNERS THE WORLD OVER TELL YOU HOW THEY FIND TIME TO RUN REGULARLY DESPITE THEIR BUSY LIVES …

'As a full-time working mother of two gymnastics-mad daughters, life can be really hectic. However, I'm a great believer in making time to exercise, which is why **I've often been on the treadmill at the gym before I reach my desk in the morning!** I've also made running a huge part of my social life: twice a week I meet my running buddy in a local park for a lunchtime run and a chat, and even at weekends I head off with other running friends for a train-as-we-talk catch-up.'
Belinda Carroll, 51, administrator, Croydon

'I love running **in the park at lunchtime** because it gives me a regular update of the seasons – in spring the daffodils and ducklings appear, in summer the tourists, then in autumn I watch the groundsmen blowing the leaves away. And winter brings the rain and snow.'
Alex Crowe, 29, IT support, London

'My job with the police means I work different shifts, so I have to fit my running around them. I find that **going for a run outside in the fresh air and daylight really helps my head to clear and my body to adjust to waking and sleeping at different times** depending on whether I'm on an early shift or night duty. And I also find the variation in the times of day I run stops it becoming a monotonous routine.'
Sophie Easton, 33, crime scene examiner, the Metropolitan Police, Surrey

'I always run in the morning as it's the only time I can regularly fit it into my day. Trouble is, I'm not a morning person, so motivating myself to get out will always be a trial. But two years on and I'm now training for a half marathon, proving that the sense of achievement I get when I've finished a run is worth even the most procrastinated and painful process of dragging myself out of the door in the first place. What I love about running is that it requires minimal equipment – all I need is a pair of trainers and I'm good to go – **I even ran in my pyjama bottoms once to save suitcase space on holiday!** There's no-one to judge me if I don't do it right and it will always be totally up to me how much I want to do and how far I want to push myself.'
Katie Froggatt, 39, PR, London

I've been **running to and from work** for about 30 years as it's the easiest way to make sure I fit running into my day. I've only forgotten to take in clothes to change into about twice – and on one of those occasions, a sympathetic cleaner lent me his tie for the day!'
John Collins, 66, manager, Swansea

'The time that works for me is **straight after work**. I get changed at the salon, then go and run in Hyde Park. If I go home first and tell myself I'll run later in the evening, I always get distracted, start eating and make excuses not to go.'
Maria O'Keefe, 32, hair salon creative director, London

'When I'm on a long car journey, rather than have a coffee break sitting in a service-station café, **I always plan my route so I can stop off and find a place like a park where I can run** – even if it's just for 15 minutes. The oxygen burst makes me feel much less tired and more relaxed for the second half of the journey.'
Michael Whalley, 62, teacher, Essex

'I decided to make my long commute home more interesting by **running to the nearest Tube station.** It felt hard at first but after a few weeks I needed a new challenge and so ran to the next station on, before catching the Tube home from there. Then I began to add one Tube stop (about 1.6K/1 mile) to my run every week. Some day soon I'll be running all the way home (which is 21K/13.1 miles) – the equivalent of a half-marathon!'
Elizabeth Gowing, 29, education consultant, London

'My job takes me all around the world, and **I throw my running gear into my suitcase even before my suit.** If I don't, I know I'll get that jittery feeling when 12 hours of sitting on the plane followed by eating way too much toxic restaurant food begin to make me crazy enough to want to run up the down escalator, slam-dance in the subway, anything to feel that endorphin high I get after a good run. When you're going insane in your hotel room and can't find a map, look in the phone book. A recent stay in the USA initially looked dismal, but the Yellow Pages revealed a park with many miles of riverside trails just beyond ugly industrial buildings.'
Randy Brophy, 45, IT consultant, Sydney, Australia

DO YOU WANT TO LEARN HOW TO MAKE EVERY RUN EASIER, MORE ENJOYABLE AND BRILLIANT FUN? WE'VE ROAD-TESTED ADVICE FROM DOZENS OF TOP EXPERTS AND ENTHUSIASTIC RUNNERS TO BRING YOU THE 101 BEST-EVER RUNNING TIPS OF ALL TIME!

7. GET THE TOP TIPS

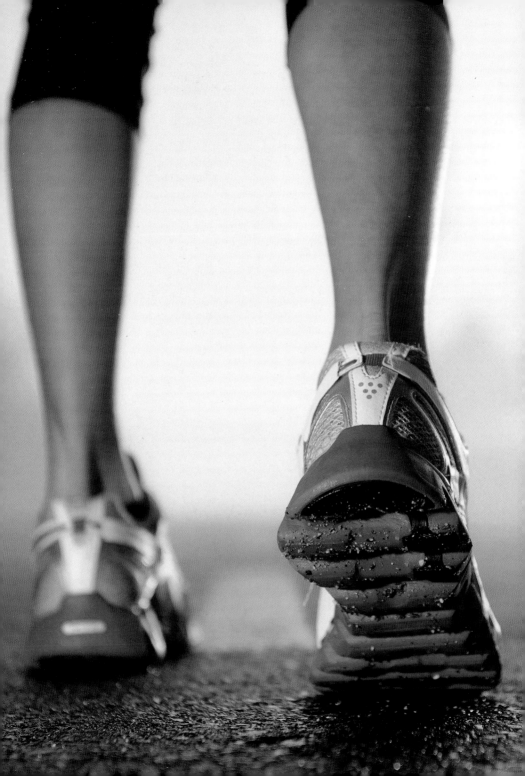

FOOD & DRINK TIPS

▶▶

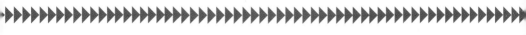

1. Don't panic!

You might think that if you take up running you have to junk whatever's in your cupboards and adopt a weird diet that revolves around endless pasta and sports drinks. Rest assured this isn't the case, especially when you're first starting out, says sports nutritionist Janet Thomson. 'As a beginner, you don't need to make radical changes to your diet, you just need to make sure you eat healthily and drink enough water,' she says. (However, if you really get bitten by the bug and start running like mad, you'll need to make some dietary changes, which we've covered in later tips.) So what counts as a healthy diet for total beginners? According to dietitian and nutritionist Dr Sarah Schenker, a healthy diet is a balanced one. 'One third of your intake should be made up of fruit and vegetables, one third made up of starchy carbohydrates (like pasta, potatoes, rice, breakfast cereals and bread) and then the remaining third should be divided up into three slices,' she explains. 'The largest slice (about 15%) should be milk and low-fat dairy foods, the second largest (about 12%) should be protein foods, such as meat, fish and vegetarian alternatives such as tofu, beans, pulses and eggs, and the final littlest slice (about 6%) should be left over for 'naughty' foods that are higher in fat and sugar – chocolate, sweets and fizzy drinks all fall into this category.' Don't struggle to split every single meal precisely into these categories – the important thing is to achieve this kind of balance over a day, a week or a lifetime!

2. Lose weight without trying

Get ready to make friends with food. Lots of people find that when they start running, they start making healthier eating choices, too. 'Taking up running gave me a natural push to think about changing my eating habits,' says Angela Charlemagne, 30, a graphic designer from London. 'I cut back loads on alcohol and fatty foods and instead started to eat more pasta, rice, fruit and veg. I lost about 3kg (7lb), and treated myself to a tasty pair of size 12 jeans to celebrate!'

3. What to eat more of

While you don't have to change all your old habits, there are certain foods that are especially great for runners, and which you might like to start mixing into your diet. Below is a list of ten favourites from Liz Applegate, a sports nutritionist at the University of California, Davis, USA.

THE TOP 10 RUNNER'S FOODS

- Wild salmon

- Lean red meat

- Tofu

- Eggs

- Broccoli

- Wholegrain bread and pasta

- Sweet potatoes

- Chicken

- Black beans

- Brown rice

4. Drink plenty

Water is wonderful – make this your mantra and you can't go wrong as a new runner. Your body needs water for just about every function it has to perform, so making sure you begin your new running programme well hydrated will help get you feeling ready for anything! Here are some ways get you into the habit of drinking plenty each day ...

▶▶ I make sure I have a big glass of water first thing in the morning before I even have breakfast or start the school run,' says keen runner and mother of three Liza Robinson, 38, from Surrey. 'This helps jog my memory to keep drinking all day long – I can easily get so busy that I forget to drink completely.'

▶▶ Buy a big bottle of water or fill a water jug and keep it on your desk so it reminds you to drink – take it to work meetings, too.

▶▶ Drink little and often. Take sips in between phone calls or every time you come back to sit at your desk.

▶▶ Fill smaller water bottles to keep with you during the day.

▶▶ Be aware of how you feel when you've drunk plenty, so you really tap into the benefits. The chances are that you're clearer headed, more alert and more energetic.

▶▶ Use the Pee Test to gauge how hydrated you are: if you've been drinking enough, your urine should be pale and odourless. The darker and smellier it becomes, the more dehydrated you are.

KNOW YOUR CARBS

▶▶

For your pre-run meal Try a chicken, prawn, tuna or cheese sandwich on granary bread, a jacket potato or granary toast with baked beans or tuna, a portion of sushi, or pasta with vegetables and tomato sauce, followed by yogurt or a handful of dried fruit such as apricots.

For your pre-run snack If your last meal was more than 4 hours ago, have a high-carb snack half an hour before your run to give you a fast energy boost. Try a slice of toast with honey or peanut butter, a handful of dried fruit and nuts or a banana.

During your run If you'll be running for longer than 60 to 90 minutes, drink an isotonic sports drink (see Tip 11), otherwise stick to water.

After your run If you're going to run quite hard again the next day, snack within 30 minutes of finishing. Consider milk-based drinks, a banana with yoghurt, a handful of nuts and dried fruit, or a flapjack with milk. In any case, eat a meal within 2–4 hours, making it a good balance of carbs and protein. Try potatoes or brown rice with meat, fish, lentils, pulses or tofu and vegetables.

5. Eat carbs for energy

Carbohydrates are a runner's best friend because they're vital for giving you enough energy to exercise. As Shelly Vella, 37, marathon runner and fashion and style director of British *Cosmopolitan* magazine puts it, 'You can't run on empty – you only get back what you put in, which means it's so important to eat right. While I'm out running, I always take a banana with me in case I get hungry, and I always really look forward to my jacket potato when I get home.' Above are suggestions for which types of carb-based meals to eat and when, from nutritionist Clare Dodgshon of the Nutrition Matters Consultancy in London.

6. Experiment!

Although expert guidelines say you should eat a meal 2–4 hours before exercise, in reality, what works best can vary from person to person, says sports nutritionist Janet Thomson. 'I'd rather exercise an hour after eating than risk feeling hungry, because then I just can't function,' she says. However, runner and sports PR consultant Jane Cowmeadow, 39, is just the opposite. 'I'm definitely someone who can't eat much before a run,' she says. 'I train every Saturday morning at 11am, and only have a couple of digestive biscuits and a mug of tea an hour or two beforehand, then save myself for a big brunch afterwards.' If you can't eat a pre-exercise meal then a healthy snack 30–60 minutes before setting out will provide the same benefits.

7. Bring a bottle

After slipping into a good sports bra and trainers, your next don't-go-running-without-it essential is a little bottle of water to hold in your hand. Plain water is all you need for any run that's less than an hour long – and current advice is to drink when thirsty rather than force yourself to drink. 'There are no hard and fast rules about how much to drink, but for most conditions 400–800ml per hour will prevent dehydration as well as overhydration' says top sports nutritionist Anita Bean. If your event or workout is longer than 30 minutes it is a good idea to drink a sports drink. The added carbohydrate and electrolytes speed absorption of fluids and have the added benefit of energy fuel and electrolytes. But don't fall into the trap of drinking excessive amounts of water, as this can bring on a potentially very dangerous condition called hyponatremia or water intoxication, when your blood is diluted so much that sodium levels fall, making you feel dizzy and causing breathing problems. Some longer-distance, slower runners in particular can tend to take in huge amounts of water and then end up collapsing after a race. You need to realize that drinking too much can be as problematic as drinking too little.

8. Eat more antioxidants

One of the very, very few drawbacks of exercise is that it increases your production of free radicals, which are unstable molecules that rampage around your body causing harm to healthy cells. Luckily, there's an easy way to fight back – by eating more antioxidant-rich foods, which are not only delicious but disarm the nasty free radicals, rendering them harmless. Below is a top-ten list of favourites complied by US-based sports nutritionist Liz Applegate.

THE TOP 10 ANTIOXIDANT FOODS AND DRINKS

- Blueberries
- Green or black tea
- Tomatoes
- Red wine (in moderation)
- Strawberries
- Pomegranate juice
- Carrots
- Spinach
- Oily fish
- Dried apricots

9. Befriend your bowels

If you're someone who suffers from constipation, here's the good news – running is an amazing, drug-free solution that should help get things moving again! But be warned, some people find running shakes things up a bit too much, making them need to go to the loo suddenly and urgently while they're out running (something that's affectionately known as getting 'runner's trots'). The good news is that this doesn't have to put you off. Here are some coping strategies ...

▶▶ Start by running somewhere with public toilets so you can gauge the effect that running has on you. After a couple of weeks, you'll know what to expect – and when! 'I always need the loo 20 minutes into a run, and then once I've been, I'm absolutely fine for the rest of the time,' says one runner. 'I just need to make sure my first loop of the park ends up outside the Ladies!'

▶▶ Experiment with what you eat beforehand – lots of runners find high-fibre cereal causes problems before an early morning run, and are better off just having toast, or running on an empty stomach. 'If I had cereal with milk before a run, I'd always end up having to call my boyfriend to come and get me in the car and whizz me home to the loo,' says one novice runner who found dairy products a particular trigger.

▶▶ Try a cup of tea or coffee to help get your bowels moving before you set off on your run.

10. Eat for recovery

If you plan to run again within 24 hours it is important to eat within 30 minutes to keep muscle soreness at bay and improve performance. Both carbohydrates and protein are essential to replenish fuel stores and help the growth and repair of muscle tissue. You should aim for snacks that contain 20g (⅔oz) of protein to maximize the recovery process. If you can't face eating straight after a run, introduce fluids to your recovery strategy. A good snack could be a chicken or lean meat sandwich, a glass of milk or flavoured milk, a hot chocolate, a milkshake or a yoghurt-based smoothie. See page 97 for more top snack ideas.

11. How to go further

If you want to start running for longer than about 60–90 minutes, carbohydrate becomes an important part of your nutrition strategy as there's a higher risk of depleting your carbohydrate (glycogen) stores,' says Anita Bean. 'This can result in early fatigue and slower performance. Consuming carbohydrate either in the form of a drink or as food provides your muscles with a ready supply of blood glucose for immediate energy, which spares glycogen stores and helps you to train longer. This should help delay fatigue and increase your endurance. For maximum performance, aim to consume 30–60g of carbohydrate per hour, depending on how hard you are exercising. That's equivalent to 400–800ml of a 6% drink (6g sugar per 100ml) such as cordial or squash diluted 1 to 6, or an isotonic sports drink.'

Chia seed is an ancient super food that is currently experiencing a renaissance. A member of the sage family, these little seeds were once a staple of the Incan, Mayan and Aztec cultures. 'Chia' is actually the Mayan word for strength and the seeds were used by these ancient cultures as an energy food, especially for their messengers, who travelled on foot and would carry a small pouch of seeds with them. You can sprinkle the seeds on salads and add them to cereals, or you can soak them in water or fruit juice and blend them with fruit to make smoothies.

12. Go-faster foods

Want to discover a secret ingredient that can help you to run faster? Then try omega-3 fatty acids. They're a type of essential fatty acid most of us really don't get enough of, but which improve the delivery of oxygen to our body's cells, increasing our energy levels and stamina. Get the right amount by eating one portion of oily fish such as mackerel, herrings, sardines, salmon or fresh tuna every week (pregnant women should limit consumption of tuna owing to the mercury it contains). One omega-3-enriched egg (Columbus eggs) or a medium-sized sweet potato will also meet your daily needs. Or try having two tablespoons of omega-3-rich linseeds with your normal bowl of cereal every morning. Soak them in a little water overnight to make it easier for your body to absorb their goodness, and then add the seeds with the water to your cereal. Alternatively, try chia seeds (see left) – mix up to three heaped tablespoons into your porridge daily.

THE TOP 10 RUNNER'S SNACKS

- Banana

- Low-fat yoghurt and piece of fruit

- Toast with peanut butter

- Fruit smoothie made with milk or yoghurt

- 2–3 fresh medjool dates

- Slice of fruit loaf or malt loaf

- Handful of dried fruit – raisins, apricots, figs, tropical-fruit mix

- Milk or milkshake or hot chocolate

- Flapjack

- Porridge with milk

13. Create a snack stash

It's almost impossible to motivate yourself to go out running if you're hungry before you even start. Squirrel away some healthy treats so you've always got a little something to eat before a run – and keep snacks to hand when you finish so you don't end up starving and miles from your next meal. See above for some great and tasty options, as recommended by accredited sports dietitian Jacqueline Boorman ...

14. Swig from the start

If you're running a longer race like a half- or full marathon, start drinking your sports drink in the early to mid part of the race – not just as the finish line comes into sight! This will give it the 20 or so minutes it needs to raise your blood-sugar levels and give you a much-needed energy burst.

15. Eat to beat injuries

Don't just eat for energy – eat to beat aches and pains, as well. The foods below can help to keep you supple and injury free:

▶▶ **Antioxidant-rich foods**
You need good supplies of foods rich in the antioxidant vitamins C and E, because studies have found they help banish post-workout soreness faster. They work their magic by battling against the nasty free radicals that are produced after exercise, and which cause muscle soreness. Getting your five portions of fruit and vegetables a day will keep your antioxidant levels nice and high, as will eating certain other foods (see Tip 8), but you can also top yours up with a good antioxidant supplement.

▶▶ **Omega-3-rich foods**
These earn another brownie point for their anti-inflammatory properties, and help both to prevent injuries and speed healing, says Anita Bean (see Tip 12 for good sources).

16. Get steamy

Steam rather than boil your veggies – it'll help to conserve more of the vitamins, minerals and precious antioxidants your body needs when you're a runner.

FIT KIT TIPS

▶▶▶

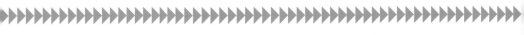

26. Let's go shopping

So you're in a sports shop and your credit card's burning a hole in your pocket – what do you need to know?

▶▶ There are two important things to look out for when choosing running gear – comfort and moisture management. Clothing should be comfortable and well tailored so that loose pieces of material don't flap or catch. For moisture management, choose a fabric such as Nike's Dri-FIT, Adidas's Climacool and Reebok's PlayIce, which "wick" (draw) sweat away from your body so it can evaporate, thus keeping you dry.

▶▶ If your thighs rub together and wear holes in your running shorts when you run, slip into something more comfortable – Lycra! One runner we know was getting through a pair of shorts every three months until she switched to Lycra – she has now had the same ones for years. (An oversized T-shirt will cover any lumpy bits the Lycra may reveal.)

▶▶ If you sweat heavily, seek out sportswear containing a new antibacterial fibre called X-STATIC. This contains pure silver, which kills 99.9% of odour-causing bacteria. X-STATIC also draws sweat away from your skin and is thermo-regulating, so it'll keep you warm in winter and cool in summer.

27. Feet first

Choosing the correct trainers is the single most important decision you'll make in your running career. Get it right and you'll be protected against injury and enjoy hundreds of miles of pain-free, smooth running. Get it wrong and you'll be exposing yourself to all sorts of problems. Here's some advice on making the right choice:

▶▶ Always go to a specialist running shop, not a high-street fashion store. You need expert advice, not the trainers being worn by the latest boy band.

▶▶ The best time of day to go shoe shopping is in the afternoon, after you've been walking about, because your feet will be at their biggest then.

▶▶ Take along any trainers you've been running in (they may help the salesperson assess your running style), as well as the socks you'll be wearing to run.

▶▶ Shoe shopping shouldn't be done in a rush. Try on lots of different trainers so you can get a good feel for what's most comfortable. Buy only trainers that feel totally comfortable from the word go, or you'll have miles of misery trying to wear them in.

▶▶ Don't skimp on what you spend. Running is a very inexpensive sport (there are no gym fees to pay and you need minimal equipment), so you can afford to splash out a bit on your trainers.

28. Insole searching

Orthotics (also known as orthoses) are thin, sole-like inserts that you slip into your trainers to iron out any kinks in the way your feet function in order to help you run more efficiently. For example, an orthotic can help stabilize your foot and ankle, or if one leg is longer than the other, it can be used to 'lengthen' your shorter leg.

Who needs orthotics? 'They're only vital for about 10% of people,' says Simon Costain, a podiatrist at The Gait & Posture Centre in Harley Street, London, 'but about 75% of people could also benefit from using them. If you develop a running injury that won't go away even though you've been to see a physio, you may find it helpful to see a podiatrist who will watch you move to determine whether your injury stems from a biomechanical imbalance and can be put right with some expert advice and the use of orthotics.' To find a podiatrist near you, visit www.feetforlife.org.

29. Test yourself

Although staff at a specialist running shop will be highly trained and ready to help you select your perfect running shoe, it's also a good idea (and quite fun) to get to know your feet beforehand, so you go in with a rough idea of the kind of shoes you should be buying. The Wet-Footprint Test, opposite, is a low-tech way to help you work out which type of trainers are most likely to suit you.

THE WET-FOOTPRINT TEST

▶▶

Step out of the bath or shower on to a piece of cardboard or a dark towel, then compare the imprint you leave with those below ...

You have a ...	So you're likely to be ...	So choose ...
Normal / neutral foot 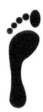	**A normal pronator**, in other words, your foot lands on the outer side of your heel and then rolls slightly inwards before you push off on the ball of your foot and your toes. This means your foot is a good shock-absorber	Trainers in the **stability** category
Flat foot 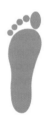	**An overpronator**, in other words, your foot lands on the outer side of your heel but then rolls inwards (or pronates) too much before you push off on the ball of your foot and your toes, which can lead to running injuries	Trainers in the **motion-control** category
High-arched foot 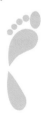	**A supinator**, in other words, your foot lands on the outer side of your heel but doesn't roll inwards enough before you push off on the ball of your foot and your toes. This means your foot isn't a very good shock-absorber	Trainers in the **cushioned** category

47. Make it sn-appy

Apps for running are available in abundance on phones, iPods and other devices – so whether you want to find new routes, improve your cadence or log your stats, there is an app for you. Examples include VIA, Bupa Smart Runner, Runtastic, Runkeeper, Strava Run, Runnit, Nike+ and Endomondo.

48. Hit the bottle

Running shops stock all manner of water bottles (plus rucksacks and belts to carry them in), so take your pick. Make sure you can run entirely comfortably holding one and that you wash it frequently in hot, soapy water. If you don't like carrying water with you, make sure you've noted where all the likely watering points are on your intended route (water fountains, taps, public toilets, pubs).

49. Be bright

Making yourself visible to passing traffic is the secret to a happy road-running career. If you're running in the dark, wear light-reflective clothes and shoes like Stewart Granby, 45, an accounting manager from Shorashim in Israel. 'Running round the city streets at night is a dangerous pastime,' he says. 'Many Israeli drivers are very impatient and no one, not even poor, defenceless runners, will stop them from getting to their final destination in the shortest possible time. At night I wear a light-coloured vest and a reflective strip across my chest and back. I'm very alert when I run and make sure I'm always aware of what the traffic's doing.'

50.
Baby, it's cold outside

There are just three things you have to remember when running in the cold: layers, layers, layers. It's far easier to remove a layer and tie it round your waist than it is to run home to fetch one! Here are some tips on how to layer up.

▶▶ **Upper body** You may need up to three layers:
Inner layer This needs to be a breathable fabric, such as Nike's Dri-FIT, Adidas's Climacool or Reebok's Playdry, which wicks (draws) moisture away from your skin and keeps you dry.
Middle layer Only necessary if it's really freezing – try wearing a fleece.
Outer layer Protects you from the elements. Try jackets with taped seams in breathable fabrics such as GORE-TEX.

▶▶ **Hands** Thin gloves made from wicking fabrics or cotton will keep your fingers toasty.

▶▶ **Legs** Your legs are very effective at generating their own heat, which means a single layer is usually adequate, but double up if you need to. Again, look for snug-fitting bottoms made from wicking fabrics.

▶▶ **Head** You lose vast amounts of heat from your head, so keep it covered with a hat.

51.
Watch it!

There is a huge array of fancy watches on the market but if you're a beginner, steer clear of any that demand a computing degree (or savvy seven-year-old!) to operate them. All you really need to follow our programme is a stopwatch feature. Another useful feature is a lap counter, which allows you to see how fast you've run every lap, mile or kilometre. You'll be using your watch on the trot, so choose one with buttons that are large enough to press with gloved fingers and big numbers that are easy to see at a glance. Watches that light up in the dark are also essential on night runs.

When it comes to investing in a GPS-enabled fitness watch, the sky's the limit in terms of price, so borrow a few from friends to help you decide what features you really need – and help you determine which brands are straightforward to use. Lisa swears by her trusty Forerunner 110 which simply tells her how far, how long and how fast she's running. It also has a heart-rate monitor that she almost never uses! There's virtually no set-up required, so you can just press 'start' and run or walk with it.

TECHNIQUE TIPS

▶▶

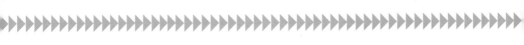

52. How to burn fat

All kinds of running burn serious calories and fat, which makes it one of the very best exercises for helping you lose weight. However, harder, higher-intensity running will help you burn more fat than easier, lower-intensity running, says top sports nutritionist Anita Bean. 'This is because it burns more calories overall per session,' she says, 'and the more calories you burn, the more fat you break down. It also keeps your metabolism speeded up for longer after you've finished, so you carry on burning calories and fat even when you're back home.' Don't panic if you think you can't do high-intensity running, though – what feels like an easy jog to one person might be high intensity to another. It's all about setting your own personal levels, and finding what represents easy and difficult sessions for you (for more on this, see Tip 59). Just make sure you mix in those harder sessions with easier ones so that you stay safe and injury free and don't get discouraged – remember that every single run, whether it's fast or slow, is a massive step along the road towards a leaner, fitter, healthier you. The key thing is to get out there and enjoy yourself.

53. Warm up well

When you're embarking on a run, don't just tear out of the front door at full pelt towards your local park. According to running expert Suzy Fitt of FittLife (www.fittlife.com), who's a tutor for British Athletics, the best way to get the most out of your training run is to prepare your body and mind with an effective dynamic warm-up. You may still see some runners holding stretches before a race or session but static stretching (holding a stretch for a period of time) is old school and it's no longer considered best practice to include it in your warm-up. Research has shown that it actually *reduces* muscle efficiency. Not to mention that if you're doing a stationary stretch, your body is cooling down and not warming up!

So what does the 'modern' so-called 'dynamic warm-up' involve? 'Begin with 5 minutes of walking or very slow running which will start to warm up your muscles, raise your heart rate, increase blood flow and focus your mind,' says Fitt. 'After a few minutes, introduce a range of rhythmic and dynamic movements (see below) to mobilize your joints and take your muscles through a full range of movement.'

Technique tips: It's important to keep your body in alignment, back straight, shoulders square and your abs engaged. Start off with small movements and gradually increase the range of movement.

1. High knees

This exercise will warm up your hip flexors, which drive your hips up and forwards during running. While running slowly, start to lift each knee a little higher. If this feels comfortable, continue to raise them until you're creating a right angle at the hip. Repeat for 30 seconds.

2. Heel flicks

Excellent for warming up your hamstrings and lightly stretching your quadriceps (the back and front of your thighs). Continue to run slowly and then start to bring your heels towards your buttocks. Gradually bring your heels higher until (if comfortable) they're touching your buttocks with each flick. Repeat for 30 seconds.

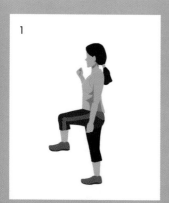

1

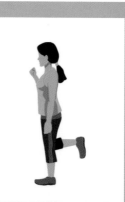

2

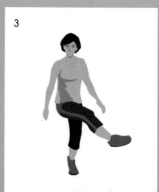

3

3. Side leg swings

Side-to-side movement is important to activate the inner- and outer-thigh muscles that help stabilize you when running. Stand tall and swing your right leg to the left diagonally across your body (as if you were trying to kick a football to a player at your left) and then swing it back and out to the right in a straight line, away from your body. Hold onto a wall if you need to. Do 10 on each leg.

4. Walking lunges

These target all the muscles you use when running. Take a big step forwards with your right leg. Keeping your body upright and central, lower your body towards the ground by bending your knees. Ensure your back is straight and that your right knee doesn't go beyond your right toe. Now bring your body back up and your feet together by stepping forwards with your left leg. Repeat by leading with your left leg. Do 10 on each leg.

5. Squat to calf raises

This exercise works the major thigh and buttock muscle groups as well as your calves. Lower yourself into a squat position by pushing your bottom out and bending at the knees (as if you're about to sit in a chair). Keep your heels firmly on the ground and ensure your knees don't go beyond your toes. Squeeze your buttocks to return to the upright position and then continue to rise up onto your toes to work your calves. Lower back down into a squat and repeat 10 times.

6. Arms and shoulders

Don't forget about your upper body. Your arms play a vital role in driving your body forwards.

- Roll your shoulders back 10 times and then forwards 10 times.
- Now place your hands out to the sides and start with small circles (pictured below) and increase until your arms are brushing your ears.
- Next, with your arms bent at right angles, drive your elbows back and forwards, gradually speeding up as if you're sprinting.
- Finally, relax and shake out your arms and shoulders.

4
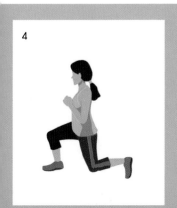

5
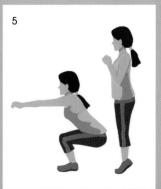

6
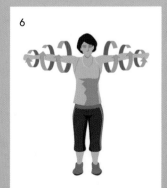

54. Wonderful warm-downs

'Going from running flat out to a dead standstill can have serious health implications as well as potentially limiting how well your body recovers,' says running expert Suzy Fitt. 'It's important to gradually lower your heart rate by reducing your pace in the last 5 minutes or more of your run. Once you feel your heart rate dropping and your breathing ease, walk briskly for a minute or two until you're fully recovered. Then carry out these five essential stretches. Post-exercise stretches are designed to realign the muscle fibres and bring your muscle length back to its pre-exercise state. Hold each stretch for up to 15 seconds on each leg. Breathe deeply and slowly when stretching. You should feel a tension in the targeted muscle – but no pain. If you experience pain or cramping, ease off the stretch. Practise your stretches with a friend so can you help each other to maintain the correct posture.

1. Upper-calf stretch

Place your hands against a support, extend your right leg backwards and gently push your right heel into the ground. Keeping your ankles, hips and shoulders in alignment, lean forwards to allow your right calf to stretch. Keep your left leg slightly bent and relaxed. Swap legs.

2. Lower-calf stretch

Ease out of the upper-calf stretch (described above) and bring your right leg in a little. Allow your right knee and ankle to bend as you lower your hips over your right foot. Ensure your right heel remains firmly on the floor. Your left foot is just for support. While keeping this position, gently push your hips forwards until you feel a stretch in the lower part of your right calf and your Achilles-tendon area. Swap legs.

3. Back-of-thigh stretch

Facing a low step or bench, place the heel of your right foot onto it while keeping your left knee slightly bent. Lean forwards slightly at the waist and push your bottom out until you feel a stretch down the back of your right thigh. Swap legs.

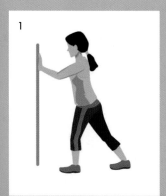
1

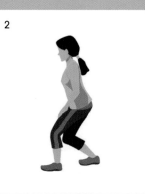
2

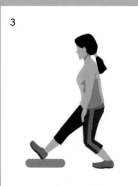
3

4. Front-of-thigh stretch

Standing up straight (holding onto a support, if necessary), bend your left knee and grasp hold of your left foot behind you. Use your left hand to ease your foot towards your left buttock, keeping your thighs and knees together. Ensure your right leg is slightly bent and your back is straight. To increase the stretch, gently push your hips forwards. Swap legs.

5. Bottom stretch

Lie on your back with your knees bent and your feet on floor. Take your left ankle and place it on your right knee. Grasp hold of your right thigh and draw it towards your chest. Feel the stretch in your bottom and outer left thigh. Swap legs.

55. Try a treadmill

It's a great idea for anyone who belongs to a gym to mix sessions on the treadmill with running outdoors, especially in the winter when the weather is bleak! Treadmills are handy as they have a display that allows you to track exactly how fast and how far you're running, and they're also soft on your knees and other joints. To build up your confidence, always start the machine up slowly and raise your speed gradually. Experiment with setting the treadmill at a 1% to 2% uphill slope to mimic what it's like to run outdoors.

56. Massage made easy

'If you're injury-prone, rub your calves with some oil before your run,' says Tim Hutchings, race director of the Brighton Marathon. 'It brings blood to the area and starts to loosen things up.'

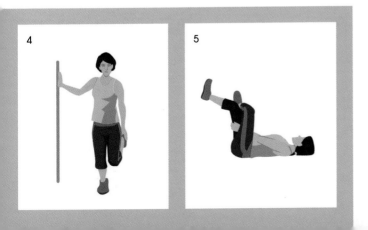

4

5

57. Be style conscious

Everyone has their very own unique running style and you shouldn't try to change yours too much without having an expert watch and advise. There are some general tips you can follow that should help you get the most out of every run you do, says Graham Anderson, a sports physio at Balance Performance Physiotherapy in London. 'Use whichever tips feel natural from the list below,' he says, 'and forget those that feel unnatural – that's probably a sign that they're wrong for you.'

▶▶ Don't hold your head too far back or forwards – to keep it in the right spot, imagine you're trying to keep a bean bag balanced on top of it.

▶▶ Keep your eyes looking ahead, not down, and your face and jaw relaxed.

▶▶ Your whole body should be upright, leaning neither forwards nor back, and your shoulders should stay relaxed. Don't let them hunch up.

▶▶ Don't swing your arms across your chest when you run as this will cause your torso to sway from side to side, which wastes precious energy that could be better used in propelling you forwards. Keep your arms relaxed and close to your body (what British Athletics calls a 'pockets to sockets' arm action, as your elbow sockets should brush your pockets). Want to go faster or tackle a hill? Focus on driving your arms backwards, as if you're trying to hammer something into a wall behind you with your elbows.

▶▶ Keep your hands loose and never clench them into fists as this can send tension snaking up your arms and into your shoulders; imagine holding something delicate between your thumb and forefinger.

▶▶ Push your hips forwards and keep your bottom tucked in rather than stuck out as you run. To get the right position, imagine you're facing a wall and trying to get your hips to touch it. At all costs, avoid running as if you're sitting in a bucket.

▶▶ Don't try to lift your knees too high unless sprinting. Think instead about driving each knee forwards, not upwards, with each stride.

58. Brilliant bows

Tie your laces in a double bow before every run to stop them coming undone when you're up and running. Having to stop mid run or, worse still, mid-race, to tie a trailing lace is just so annoying.

59. Six successful running sessions

One of the brilliant things about running is that it can be whatever you want it to be – easy or hard, fast or slow, competitive or fun. If running at the same speed over the same distance every time you go out is what suits you, that's great, and you're certainly not doing anything wrong. If, on the other hand, this leaves you feeling a little bored, then there are all sorts of different running sessions you might want to try in order to burn more calories, boost your fitness, get you ready for a race, or simply keep you feeling motivated, challenged and raring to go. We asked sports scientist Joe Dunbar to help us put together this list of six super-successful sessions for you to try for size. Use them to keep your running feeling varied, but don't suddenly start doing back-to-back hard sessions – always follow every day of hard work with either a rest day or a day of easier running, so you give your body enough time to recover properly.

Base running
(aka Sunday-morning running)

Perfect for those lazy Sunday mornings, this is the most basic level of running. On a scale of 1–10, with 1 being least effort and 10 being toughest, it's sitting pretty in the middle at number 5. Pad along like this and you'll be quite capable of holding a conversation, and checking out what's going on around you. 'This is the kind of speed you'd use if you were going on a longer run, or as an easy recovery run if you'd worked harder the day before,' says Dunbar. The point of it is to build a good base level of fitness, and get your muscles accustomed to taking up and using oxygen and burning fat as fuel.

Steady-state running
(aka running-late-for-Sunday-dinner pace)

This is one step on from base running – the kind of pace you'd go at if you knew you were running a touch late for that Sunday dinner with the in-laws. Although you still feel relaxed and leisurely, and you can still chat away quite well, your effort level has gone up to 7 on the scale. Learn to use this pace on some of your medium-to-long runs: 'It'll get you into a bit better condition, and also start to work your heart and lungs a little harder,' says Dunbar.

Fartlek running
(aka fun-and-frisky running)

This one's fun, fun, fun – honest! Its risqué-sounding name is in fact a Swedish word meaning speed play, and this session asks you to do just that – to play with your speed so you have fun at a variety of different paces. Your session could go a little like this: during a jaunt round the park, you might warm up, run slowly up a small hill, then put in a fast sprint down the other side (as if you'd spotted the last pair of size 6 shoes in the January sales), slow down again until you get to the next lamp-post or tree, then run fast over gently undulating ground for a minute or two, enjoying the sense of rhythm. Consequently, your effort levels will also vary – from 8 or 9 when you're running fast, back down to 5 as you recover. 'Fartlek is a means of getting your body used to running and working at different speeds,' says Dunbar. 'It's a great way to have your first go at running faster because it's so unstructured – you can simply do what you feel capable of. Think of it as the come-and-have-a-go session.' You can make it feel even more fun by doing it with friends, but do be warned: if you're attempting to do it in the street, you may look a lot less dignified than those base-level Sunday runners!

Tempo running
(aka gets-you-gasping running)

If we're honest, you might not exactly look forward to this type of session, but it's great if you want to bring your running on in leaps and bounds. That's why it's probably best if you do it once you're starting to feel fitter rather than in your first week of entering into the wonderful world of running. On a tempo run your effort level has gone up to 8, you're now breathing hard, and your chat has been left behind as you can only just manage to squeeze out a few words when you're running like this. Which means it actually feels pretty tough. So why bother to put yourself through all this? Because it's a brilliant way to burn calories, work your heart and lungs, and boost your fitness without having to run for hours on end. 'Run like this and you'll be getting the very best aerobic workout,' says Dunbar. 'And, although it sounds like hard work, it's actually great for lazy runners as you don't have to go on for very long, and you can even take a break in the middle of the session!' Try it yourself by starting with a 5-minute warm-up, then doing 5 minutes of tempo running, taking a 2-minute jog break (during which time you allow your breathing and heart rate to slow a little to prepare for the next effort), then tempo running for another 5 minutes. A great workout in under 20 minutes, and you'll still have time to get to the pub before last orders.

Interval training
(aka quick-slow running)

For interval training you need a bit more inner grit and discipline, and a watch that measures seconds. What you do is alternate between timed bursts of hard running (at an effort level of 8 to 9) and timed easier 'recovery' periods (at an effort level of 2 to 4), which allow you to slow down and get your breath back. 'For your first session, try running hard for 60 seconds, then recovering at a slower pace for 60 seconds, and building up to being able to repeat this pattern eight times,' says Dunbar. The idea is to keep going at the same pace during each of your hard efforts, rather than gradually tailing off. If you find this all too hard, you can do an easier version of intervals where you work slightly less intensely in the hard effort each time (say at an effort level of 7 to 8). Again, sessions like these are great calorie burners and train your body to be able to run faster for longer periods. So when you go back to doing your normal runs, you may find yourself flying along!

Hill running
(aka 'I-will-survive' running)

Powerful and potent for your body and mind, hill running will improve your mental muscle as well as the muscles in your legs and bottom. Can you go for that promotion? You bet. Dare you ask for that pay rise? Oh yes. Once you can take on that dreaded hill, facing up to just about anything else seems easy. 'Start out gradually with just a couple of bursts of hill running, and work up to doing 8 or 10,' says Dunbar. 'Run up the hill for 20 to 30 seconds, gently jog or walk down again, then go up again, repeating the whole process eight times.' You'll also find your effort levels vary just like when you're doing intervals – between 8 to

9 on the way up the hill and between 2 and 4 on the way down again. You can choose anything from gentle to steep hills, depending on how hard on yourself you want to make it.

So, what's the point? Having to work against the upward slope of the hill challenges your body in a new way, forcing it to work harder, and it really tests your quad muscles at the front of your thighs. Doing hills will also make you feel pretty invincible. Worth trying for the mental boost alone.

60. Joint effort

If you're worried that running is giving your joints a battering, take heart from the very positive results of a study at Stanford University, California, USA. From tracking 538 runners and 423 non-runners, aged about 58, the study revealed that the runners developed disabling joint changes an average of 12 years later than the non-runners. What's more, another study of 74,000 runners, published in *Medicine & Science in Sports & Exercise*, has shown that we're actually about 50% less likely to need a hip replacement or to develop osteoporosis than walkers, most probably because of running's weight-loss benefits.

61. Trick yourself

'Lots of people have a mental block about increasing the distance that they run. If you're finding it tough, try this crafty trick,' says David Francis, 42, a fitness instructor from Oxfordshire. 'Run as far as you can comfortably go on one outing, then the next time you go out, run just one lamp-post or tree farther. It's a really easy way to increase your stamina without it feeling like a struggle.'

62. Beat jelly belly

You might think having strong legs is all that counts in running, but in fact the state of your stomach and back is pretty important, too. If they're weak, they'll tend to sag and curve as you get tired, so your body forms a sort of C-shape, making it much harder for your legs to do their work because they won't have a stable, solid platform to work from. If, however, you have a strong torso, it provides vital support for your whole body and a strong base for your legs to power from, helping you keep on running well even when you're tired.

To develop the right muscles, you need to do core-stability work (so called because it builds a strong and stable core for your whole body). Ideally, try attending Pilates classes, which work on activating not just the superficial muscles of your torso, but also the deeper ones such as the transverse abdominis, which wraps round your whole torso helping keep everything in the right place. 'And when you're out running (and simply day to day), think about tensing and engaging your stomach muscles, and drawing your tummy button towards your spine to help improve your posture and strengthen your torso,' says personal trainer Laura Williams.

63. Rest when you're ill

Don't struggle out for a run when you're feeling awful, especially if you've got a fever, as this could increase your risk of dehydration, heatstroke and even heart failure, says

71. How to stay injury-free

▸▸ Always wear good trainers and replace them every 600 miles or so.

▸▸ Warm up properly – while it may not prevent injury, it's a good idea to take your muscles and joints through a full range of movement before you start a run (see Tip 53).

▸▸ Vary the surfaces you run on to reduce impact on your joints – try to run on grass, trails and a track as well as roads and pavements.

▸▸ Be aware of any areas in your body that are tensing up while you're running and consciously try to relax them.

▸▸ Get any niggling problems seen to early by a qualified physiotherapist – neglecting aches and pains can put stress on other areas of your body.

▸▸ Don't try to take things too fast too soon and always have a rest day after a hard session.

72. Six-packs for speed

Not convinced speed-training's worth the effort? Think again. 'When I was at university,' says Loren Jackson, 44, a lawyer from Lubumbashi, Democratic Republic of Congo, 'my running club challenged any runners who hadn't previously done speed-training to try doing it once a week for a month. Anyone whose performance in a 5K (3 mile) race didn't improve as a result was promised a six-pack of beer. As far as I know, no one ever won the beer!'

73. Can you run when pregnant?

It's certainly not the time to take up running if you've never run before, but if you're fit, healthy and used to running, there's no reason why you can't keep going gently. You will need to make a few changes though, as it's important not to get totally breathless, and not to get too hot and sweaty while you're exercising. If you take the intensity of your runs down a notch and listen to what feels right for your body, then you should be able to continue enjoying your running while pregnant. Paula Radcliffe showed the way for lots of women when she took part in a 10K race – at a more gentle pace than her normal blistering one – when just over five months pregnant. Once you've given birth, speak to your GP about how soon you can start running again.

If you've not had a Caesarean or any other major complications, many doctors will tell you it's fine to run about six weeks after the birth. But again, base your decision on how your body is feeling.

74. Put your feet up

Here's one piece of expert advice we know you're going to love: to get fit it's just as important to rest as it is to run. 'When you run,' says David Castle, editor of *Men's Running* UK, 'your muscles and ligaments develop microscopic tears. This isn't a problem if you give them time to repair themselves by resting. However, if you don't give yourself time off, these tiny tears can become full-on strains and your running can suffer massively. Rest is particularly vital after speedwork sessions, hard races and long runs. The easiest way to make sure you're getting enough rest is to designate one day a week as a day when you take it really easy. Beginners should have more time off, as should older runners.' Castle also suggests you nominate one month each year as a rest month. 'Cut your overall mileage in half,' he says, 'and replace some of your regular runs with cross-training activities such as swimming, cycling or gym work. This is a great way to strengthen your body, recharge your batteries and ensure you keep enjoying every run.'

75. Perform the Rope Trick

If you think hills are hellish, try this tip used by Bruce Fordyce, the legendary South African runner who won the unbelievably hilly Comrades ultra-marathon an amazing nine times. 'When you're tackling a hill,' he says, 'imagine you're pulling yourself up it using two parallel ropes. Really power your arms but keep your hands nice and relaxed. It truly does help turn mountains into molehills.'

76. Get enough sleep

'As you start running more, you'll probably also find you need to start sleeping for longer periods,' says Professor Tim Noakes, Discovery health chair of exercise and sports science at the University of Cape Town, South Africa. 'If, for example, you run for two hours, you may well need an extra hour's sleep as well, which means you'll have to learn how to budget your time to fit in the running and extra sleeping.'

MOTIVATION TIPS

▶▶

77. Get fancy!

Want to feel like an A-list celebrity for a few hours? Fancy having crowds straining to get a glimpse of you, hearing wild cheers when you finally make your appearance, and having photographers leaping out at every bend in the road? All you have to do is enter any well-supported race, slip into a fancy-dress outfit and voilà! 'Dressing up can be tremendously motivating,' says top life coach Fiona Harrold, 'as you'll get twice as much support from the crowd, who'll really appreciate the effort you went to.' One word of warning, though: take your outfit on a few trial runs before race day or you may find your Batman cape hampers rather than hastens your progress.

78. Fib to yourself

'I have the running bug and no kind of medicine can make it go away,' says Stuart Major, 41, a policeman from Surrey. 'And yet, like most runners I know, there are times when I really don't feel like going for a run. I get home from work, I'm tired and hungry, and all I want to do is sit and watch TV. On those days I tell myself to do just 20 to 30 minutes – I'll be back before I know it. So I head out and, after 10 minutes, I usually feel much better and consider running 40 or 50 minutes. When I've finished the run, I no longer feel tired or hungry and am thrilled I managed to do it.'

97. Enter a race

Don't be intimidated by races as they can give you a massive motivation boost. They're a brilliant way of providing you with a goal, meeting other runners and assessing your progress. Plus, they're the ultimate way to make sure you stick to your training programme – the mere thought of struggling through a race because you haven't trained can be enough to spur you on to run regularly. Sharon Lindores, 35, a journalist, found this out when she moved to Edmonton in Canada, where winters are so harsh that some runners put nails on the bottom of their shoes to get better grip on icy patches! 'I found running in the dark at -40˚C (-40˚F) really hard,' she says, 'so to keep me motivated, I signed up for a spring race. Running in the winter made me feel as if I was defying the elements and, when spring finally arrived, I was in good-enough shape to do my race and enjoy longer runs in the good weather.'

A race is also a good opportunity to see places you've been dying to visit. Always wanted to zoom round Silverstone Racetrack? Potter along Charles Bridge in Prague? Run through Berlin's Brandenburg Gate? There are races that will allow you to do all these things.

98. Buddy up

Training with a running partner is a sure-fire way to make runs more fun (and frequent!). Emma Simpson, 31, a designer from Sussex, swears by running with a partner, or in her case two. 'I was determined to regain my former fitness after having my baby,' she says, 'so I talked two mums from my antenatal class into coming with me once a week while our partners looked after our children. It's hard to give yourself permission to have time off when you're a parent, but going for a run with my friends gives us time away from our partners and children and a chance to have a laugh and a natter while relaxing and getting fit.'

99. Be competitive

'Having something to aim for is essential to keep up your momentum,' says Danielle Sellwood, co-founder of Sportsister.com. 'Entering an event and adding a little bit of competition to your running can really make a difference. Choose a realistic target, such as a 5K (3 mile) race and perhaps aim to do it in, say, 35 minutes, so you have something to aim for.' Parkruns (www.parkrun.org.uk), which are free, weekly, 5K timed runs held in picturesque parks in the UK and around the world every Saturday morning, are ideal for this, as are events in the women-only Race For Life series (www.raceforlife.org). 'Having recorded a time,' says Sellwood, 'you can aim to go a little bit faster at your next event. If you continually set yourself targets and reach them, it'll really help to build your confidence.' Running more quickly isn't the only way you can be competitive: Parkruns award T-shirts to runners who've attended 10, 50, 100 and 250 events, so see if you can be the first of your friends to bag one.

100. One potato, two potato

Losing weight can be a marvellous incentive to keep running. 'Each time you lose a couple of pounds, buy the same weight in potatoes and keep them in a bag in your kitchen,' says Karen Reeve, 28, a director's PA from Somerset. 'Then, when you want to skip a run you're scheduled to do, pick up the bag and say to yourself, "Running helped me lose this much weight – do I really want to miss this session?" Those potatoes will help you realize you'd be better off going running after all.'

101. Just one last thing ...

Yes, we know we said 100 tips but we needed room for just one more! If you're feeling mind boggled by all the advice we've just given you, don't forget the most important tip of all. Running is meant to be fun. Don't get hung up on whether you're doing it right or wrong (unless it's injuring or hurting you, of course) – the more you run, the more you'll learn. In the meantime, just get out and enjoy it!

NOW YOU'RE READY TO TAKE THE
NEXT STEP AND RUN THAT LITTLE
BIT FARTHER, WE'VE DEVISED
THREE TRAINING PLANS TO SPEED
YOU ALONG. PLUS WE'VE GOT INFO
ON CROSS-TRAINING WORKOUTS TO
BOOST YOUR RUNNING POTENTIAL,
AND THE LOW-DOWN ON HOW
TO ENJOY EVERY RACE TO THE
MAXIMUM ...

8. GET EVEN BETTER

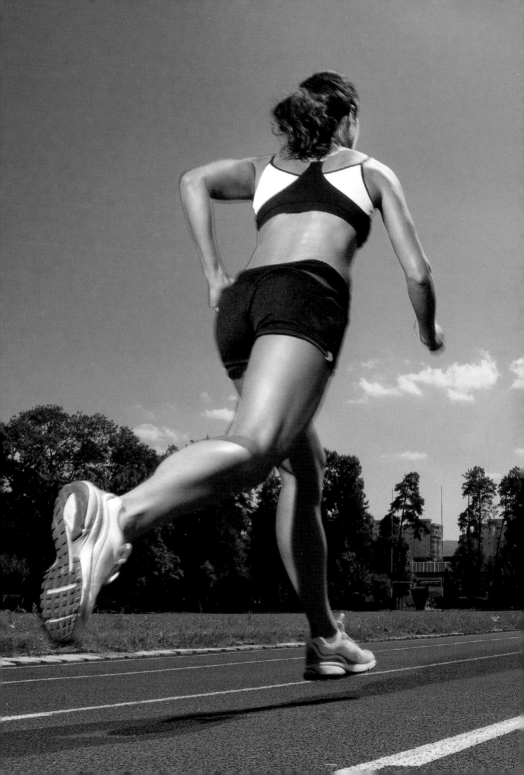

RACING AHEAD!

Want some excitement in your life? Then enter a race – you'll never look back ...

Falling in love with running is quite like settling into a new relationship – after the initial heart-racing, cheek-flushing thrill has worn off, you have to work hard to avoid slipping into the equivalent of a TV-dinner and slippers-by-the-fire comfort zone, where you stick to what you know, and do the same two laps of the park on the same three nights every week. Of course, there's nothing wrong with getting cosy and comfy with running; it's just that if you dare to challenge yourself and inject a little more excitement into your running routine, you'll get so much more fun from it. Muster the courage to take on a new challenge and you'll be repaid a hundred times over by the changes you see in not just your body but your mind, your attitude and your whole life.

GET FASTER, GO FARTHER

This chapter is dedicated to helping you improve, whether you want to start running faster or go farther. We believe the best way for you to do this is to enter a race so you have a goal to aim for. If the mere thought of this makes your knees knock with fear, don't worry – we've been there, too, and everyone has to start somewhere. Even the legendarily awesome marathon supremo Paula Radcliffe came 299th (out of 600 plus) in her first national race, and just look at her now!

GLORY AND GLAMOUR

There's nothing like the feeling of fear and anticipation as you line up with hundreds of other runners on the start line, or the glory and glamour of running towards the finish line that brings out the natural show-off in us all. To take you smoothly into your first race and beyond, we've put together three training plans that'll help you run any distance you've set your heart on. If you followed The 60-Second-Secret Plan in Chapter 6, you're already capable of doing a 5K (3 mile) race, so the plans in this chapter will help get you round a 10K (6 mile) race, a half-marathon (21K/13.1 miles) and a marathon (42.2K/26.2 miles). They're designed for you to work through in sequence, so you build up your fitness gradually, and enjoy every step. Each one follows a slightly different format as each was designed by a different expert, but they all contain principles that will be familiar to you from Chapters 6 and 7, such as walk/run sessions and tempo running. Plus we've got info on which cross-training workouts are best for runners, and tips and advice on how to get the most from them.

FIVE WAYS TO START IMPROVING – RIGHT NOW!

▶▶▶

1. Remember where you started.
If you think you can't improve, remind yourself of just how far you've already come – and then start imagining how much farther you can go.

2. Get some support
It's hard to improve all alone – run with someone who's better than you, or join a running club to provide extra motivation.

3. Race against the clock
Run with a watch and aim to keep beating your times. Try a two-lap run, on which you time your first lap, then aim to run faster on the second lap.

4. Be kind to yourself
'Push your limits,' says Lisa Buckingham, 25, a sub-editor from London, 'but never so far that you feel really awful. Your brain stores information like that, and if you start associating running with pain or feeling terrible, your motivation will melt away.'

5. Get inspired
Go along and spectate at the first race you're intending to run. It'll help you get familiar with the course and give you a good idea of what to expect on the day. But best of all, when you see the cheering crowds and how much fun everyone is having, it'll motivate you to join in.

'MY MOST MEMORABLE RACE'

TECHNICAL DIFFICULTIES, SPA BATHS AND ACHIEVING THE IMPOSSIBLE – SIX RUNNERS SHARE
THEIR FAVOURITE RACE-DAY MEMORIES ...

'When my Walkman failed just as the gun went off on the start line of a 5K
(3 mile) Race For Life, I was gutted. Listening to music was the only way I'd
learnt to run – the beat kept me at an even pace and stopped me panicking
as I couldn't hear how out of breath I was! But as people all around me surged
forwards, **I realized it was too late to chicken out, even though the last time I'd
been in a race I'd been jumping down the school field in a sack.** Those three
miles were the hardest I've ever run, but I didn't stop or slow down once. When
I finally crossed the finish line, red-faced and panting, I was ecstatic. I love
running outside now, and despite the fact that I can easily run more than three
miles, that first race was my most important achievement. My medal still
reminds me that I can do anything when I put my mind to it.'
Charlotte Stacey, 26, journalist, London

'I'll always be grateful to my first race, the Flora Light Women's Challenge, for
teaching me to run outdoors. I'd been running on the treadmill at the gym
for a couple of years but was always too shy and embarrassed to run outside.
But then I decided to do the race with my friend, and **we just treated it as a
laugh, telling each other we could stop whenever we wanted.** I loved it and
never looked back – straight after that, I started running on Clapham Common
while training for the London Marathon, and running on family weekends
away. Now I've got a dog and love going for runs in the woods with her.
It's opened up a whole new world!'
Liza Robinson, 38, physiotherapist, Surrey

'My favourite race is a half-marathon run in Ein Gedi at the Dead Sea, the
lowest point on Earth. **To your left is the Dead Sea and to your right are
the Jordean mountains, creating one of the most picturesque locations in
the world.** After the race, you can go to the spa in Ein Gedi and soak in
baths rich with salt and other minerals, making this a very relaxing and
enjoyable weekend.'
Stewart Granby, 45, accounting manager, Shorashim, Israel

'Running the Adidas Mini London Marathon (4.2K/2.65 miles) was hard but it
was **the best day of my life**! I felt I'd really achieved something.'
Leo Kellock, 12, pupil, London

'During my first race (the 16K/10 mile Great South Run in Portsmouth), I realized **running is as much about what's going on in your head as what you're doing with your body.** As I got tired in the final stages of the run, I found myself literally saying out loud, "You can do it, you can do it." I got to the finish having run the whole way and just felt so proud that I wanted to cry.'
Maria O'Keefe, 32, hair salon creative director, London

'The most emotional thing I've ever done is the Comrades Marathon, an 89K (55.6 mile) race from Pietermaritzburg to Durban in South Africa. For 16 years I watched the race on TV, from the dawn start to the final gun at dusk, and felt choked with emotion. Then, one year, I found myself shivering on the start line and couldn't hold back the tears. My fondest memory of the whole run was passing a school for handicapped kids. The tots were in calipers, on crutches, or with artificial legs, and those that could had their hands outstretched for us to high five as we ran past.

    With 28K (17.5 miles) to go, I thought I wouldn't make it before the cut-off time, but as I got closer to the finish, **all I can recall is the spectators willing us on, eager to help in any way they could,** even if it was just wiping my sunglasses clean on their dry T-shirts. At the entrance to the stadium where the race finished, I started retching but the crowd yelled, "Don't stop!" and a stranger grabbed my wrist and said, "You've got to run! Stay with me." All I could think of as I ran towards the line (and the man who fires the final gun to signal that the cut-off time has been reached and you're not allowed to finish) was, "You can't be sick here in front of the TV cameras!". As I staggered to the finish, the spectators were beside themselves, screaming us in, willing us to make it ... and I did, by 18 seconds. A few days after the race, a friend, who avoids all exercise, called me to ask how it went and said "What took you so long?"'
Pam Newby, 54, webmaster, Cape Town, South Africa

'The Hyde Park Race For Life will always hold incredibly special memories for me. It was a joy running with my marathon-mad Mum, and the last time I'd ever run a race with her because she died of cancer a year later. We did it with my six-year-old daughter and a dozen friends to celebrate my own victory over breast cancer. I loved the buzz, the laughter - but most of all, being able to run again.'
Darian Jeffs, 44, administrator, Oxford

YOUR 10K PLAN

WHO'S IT GOOD FOR?

Anyone who has run a 5K (3 mile) race and is ready to go that little bit farther – 10K is equivalent to just over 6 miles. It's a great taster race for new runners and is also ideal for speed freaks who'd rather run faster over a shorter distance, and anyone who comes out in a rash at the thought of doing a marathon.

- **How does it feel?** Lovely! It's just far enough to feel like a 'proper' race, and to allow you to test yourself, but without feeling like too much of a hard slog or meaning you have to train too hard.

- **How long will it take?** Less than 45 minutes and you're flying, about an hour is good, over an hour and you'll be in good company with the slightly more leisurely but still perfectly respectable runners.

- **What's the plan?** A 10-week programme designed by sports scientist Joe Dunbar.

Effort levels for your sessions are given in brackets, with 1 being the easiest and 10 the hardest. Don't forget to warm up before each session (see pages 116–117) and cool down and stretch (see pages 118–119) afterwards.

WEEK 1

Monday: Walk 20 mins (effort level 2–4)
Tuesday: Rest
Wednesday: Run 5 mins (effort level 5), walk 3 mins (effort level 2). Repeat once more (Total: 16 mins)
Thursday: Rest
Friday: Run 7 mins (effort level 5), walk 2 mins (effort level 2). Repeat once more (Total: 18 mins)
Saturday: Rest
Sunday: Run 15 mins (effort level 5)

WEEK 2

Monday: Walk 30 mins (effort level 2–4)
Tuesday: Rest
Wednesday: Run 10 mins (effort level 5), walk 2 mins (effort level 2–4). Repeat once more (Total: 24 mins)
Thursday: Rest
Friday: Run 7 mins (effort level 5), walk 2 mins (effort level 2–4). Repeat once more (Total: 18 mins)
Saturday: Rest
Sunday: Run 20 mins (effort level 5)

WEEK 3

Monday: Walk 30 mins (effort level 4)
Tuesday: Rest
Wednesday: Run 15 mins (effort level 6)
Thursday: Rest
Friday: Run 10 mins (effort level 5), walk 3 mins (effort level 4). Repeat once more (Total: 26 mins)
Saturday: Rest
Sunday: Run 25 mins (effort level 5)

WEEK 4

Monday: Run 15 mins (effort level 5)
Tuesday: Rest
Wednesday: Run 20 mins (effort level 5)
Thursday: Rest
Friday: Run 15 mins (effort level 7)
Saturday: Rest
Sunday: Run 30 mins (effort level 5)

WEEK 5

Monday: Run 20 mins (effort level 5)
Tuesday: Rest
Wednesday: Run 20 mins (effort level 7)
Thursday: Rest
Friday: Run 25 mins (effort level 5 to 6)
Saturday: Rest
Sunday: Run 35 mins (effort level 5)

WEEK 6

Monday: Walk 40 mins (effort level 3-4)
Tuesday: Rest
Wednesday: Run 5 mins (effort level 5),
then repeat the following 5 times:
run 1 min (effort level 8 to 9), walk
1 min (effort level 2) (Total: 15 mins)
Thursday: Rest
Friday: Run 25 mins (effort level 5-6)
Saturday: Rest
Sunday: Run 40 mins (effort level 5)

WEEK 7

Monday: Run 20 mins (effort level 5)
Tuesday: Rest
Wednesday: Run 5 mins (effort level 5),
then repeat the following 6 times:
run 1 min (effort level 8-9), walk
1 min (effort level 3-4) (Total:17 mins)
Thursday: Rest
Friday: Run 20 mins (effort level 7)
Saturday: Rest
Sunday: Run 45 mins (effort level 5)

WEEK 8

Monday: Walk 40 mins (effort level 4)
Tuesday: Rest
Wednesday: Run 5 mins (effort level 5),
then repeat the following 8 times:
run 1 min (effort level 8-9), walk
1 min (effort level 4) (Total: 21 mins)
Thursday: Rest
Friday: Run 30 mins (effort level 5-6)
Saturday: Rest
Sunday: Run 50 mins (effort level 5)

WEEK 9

Monday: Run 25 mins (effort level 5)
Tuesday: Rest
Wednesday: Run 5 mins (effort level 5),
then repeat the following 8-10 times,
depending on what you can manage:
run 1 min (effort level 8-9), run 1 min
(effort level 5) (Total: 21-25 mins)
Thursday: Rest
Friday: Run 20 mins (effort level 7)
Saturday: Rest
Sunday: Run 60 mins (effort level 5)

WEEK 10

Monday: Run 30 mins (effort level 5)
Tuesday: Rest
Wednesday: Run 20 mins (effort level 7)
Thursday: Rest
Friday: Rest
Saturday: Rest
Sunday: 10K RACE! (effort level 5-6)

HOW TO FIND YOUR PERFECT RACE

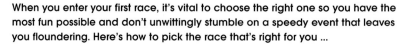

When you enter your first race, it's vital to choose the right one so you have the most fun possible and don't unwittingly stumble on a speedy event that leaves you floundering. Here's how to pick the race that's right for you ...

- **Choose your distance (from 5K to 10K to half-marathon to full marathon),** then buy a running magazine (see page 222) or browse online for race and listings. Once you've picked a race, you can usually enter it online at *Runner's World's* fab website www.runnersworld.co.uk.

- **Once you've short-listed a few races, the most important things to find out are how fast and how big the race is.** You're probably better off with a slower, bigger race the first time as in small, fast races you may find yourself bringing up the rear and running on your own. It's also good to know what the ratio of male to female runners will be (if you're a woman, it's better to enter a female-friendly race rather than going it alone with a bunch of super-competitive male club runners). The reviews on www.runnersworld.co.uk will give you unbiased views of what the race is like. Alternatively, ask someone who's already run it, or contact the race director.

- **Try to enter an event where there's lots of crowd support to encourage you when the going gets tough.** Some races are mobbed by spectators who'll stay for hours and cheer the very last runners over the finish line, others can be a bit of a lonely wasteland.

- **You also want to think about the practicalities.** Is the race easy to travel to? Will you have to stay somewhere overnight? How much will the whole thing − from race entry to transport − cost?

- **Finally, think about the goodies!** Do you get a lovely shiny medal on a pink ribbon? Are you handed a goodie bag stuffed with food and drink as you cross the finish line? Will you be given a 'been-there-run-that' souvenir T-shirt that you can proudly wear afterwards? Or do you have to make do with a pat on the back and a long walk home? After you've just run for more than half an hour, believe us, it matters!

RACE DAY CHECKLIST

▶▶

- **Race number (forget it, and forget running the race!)**
- **Safety pins**
- **Trainers (and a spare pair)**
- **Running top/vest**
- **Running jacket**
- **Running shorts/bottoms**
- **Sports bra**
- **Knickers/underpants**
- **Socks**
- **Hat**
- **Gloves**
- **Sports watch/GPS-enabled fitness watch**
- **Bin bag (to keep you warm)**
- **Fancy-dress outfit!**

- **Change of clothes plus flip-flops (great for tired feet)**
- **Kit bag**
- **Sports drink/water bottle**
- **Snacks/sweets**
- **Sunscreen**
- **Sunglasses**
- **Bumbag/mini rucksack**
- **Loo roll**
- **Vaseline**
- **Blister plasters**
- **Painkillers**
- **Cash**
- **Phone**
- **Camera**
- **MP3 player (if the race allows it – many don't)**

MIX IT UP

We thought we'd take a short break before launching into the half-marathon and marathon training plans, to tell you about the benefits of cross-training ...

Cross-training might sound a bit technical, but it's not – it's basically just a term that means including a mix of different activities in your regular fitness programme – from cycling to swimming to weight-training. Together, these combine to bring you big fitness benefits, and even better, help improve your running.

When you're a new runner and keen to improve as much as you can, as fast as you can, it's easy to think that the more you run, the better you'll get. Yet, while that's true to a certain extent, it also pays not to overdo the pavement-pounding, as it can lead to you getting injured or bored.

Which is where cross-training comes in – by adding a few different fitness activities into the mix along with your running, you can give your body a break, while working on different aspects of your fitness and strength that will complement and enhance your running. And give you great arms, a toned tummy and pert bottom in the process!

To help get you started, we asked fitness expert Jon Roberts, from Matt Roberts Personal Training (www.mattroberts.co.uk) to give us a run-down of some of the most runner-friendly cross-training activities and some tips and advice on how to make the most of each of them.

You'll never fit them all into your week, so just choose the types of cross-training that appeal the most to you and give them a go.

SWIMMING

Swimming is a great way to work your upper and lower body at the same time, and because you can do a variety of different strokes, you can choose to target different sets of muscles.

How will it help my running?

It'll work your heart and lungs, building up your stamina. Working against the resistance provided by the water is also a good way to strengthen your muscles. But, as a runner, one of the best things about swimming is that it allows you to reap these fitness benefits while giving your legs a welcome break from the impact they get during running.

Which strokes are best?

The best stroke for runners looking to build stronger muscles is front crawl, because of its powerful kicking action. To get results, you'll need to put some effort in – we've put together a good session for you to try (see Try this ... opposite).

How often do I need to do it?

A once-a-week swim alongside regular running sessions should be enough for you to feel the benefits. If you've been injured, try swimming twice a week to maintain your fitness without overdoing it, and get you ready to start running again.

You'll also find that having a lovely relaxing swim the day after a race is a blissful way to shake off your aches and stay active without overstretching yourself.

Try this ...
The best way to get the most from swimming is to work in short intervals. Try the workout below:

- Two lengths of regular front crawl, swimming at a medium/fast pace
- Two lengths of front crawl kick, using your legs only, holding a float, swimming at a fast pace
- Two lengths of front crawl using arms only, holding a float between your legs, swimming at a medium pace, with powerful strokes
- Rest for 45 seconds, then repeat

Any top tips?
- To improve your swimming, always swim with goggles. Lots of people swim with their heads out of the water, which is bad news for your neck and upper back.
- Most pools have a clock with a hand that measures seconds. Try timing yourself swimming one length and then work on beating your best time on each visit.
- You could also count how many strokes you take on a typical length, and try gradually to decrease that number by getting more power into each stroke.

CYCLING

Cycling is a fantastic aerobic activity that'll really get your heart and lungs working hard, and again will strengthen your legs without you having to do more pavement-pounding.

How will it help my running?
Cycling regularly will help you build thighs and calves of steel. It'll also build your stamina and get your heart and lungs super-fit. This is because you can cycle at a good pace on a bike without your legs getting tired too quickly, which allows you to keep your heart pumping harder and for longer periods than if you tried to sprint during a run.

What type of cycling is best?
Hill-training is a great way for runners to really strengthen their legs. Your best tactic is to find a good hill that you can tackle a few times. Try cycling up it for 5 minutes, down it for 2 minutes, and then doing it again.

If you find you get bored cycling alone, try a spinning class on static bikes at the gym. They're amazing calorie burners, and will really push your fitness to another level – just don't do one the day before a race, as you'll tire your legs out.

How often do I need to do it?
A few times a week will bring you big fitness benefits. If you struggle to fit this in, think creatively, and consider cycling to work or to the gym, or getting together with friends to make weekend cycle rides more fun.

Any top tips?

- Visit your local bike shop and ask them to check that your bike is set up properly. Lots of people ride with their saddle too low; this can feel uncomfortable and you won't get the best body benefits from your rides.
- Don't make the classic mistake of cycling along slowly in a really tough gear – you will exhaust your legs without giving your heart a good workout. Instead, cycle along faster in a lower gear, which will allow your legs to spin more freely.
- If you want to cycle longer distances regularly, consider getting a gel-filled cover for your saddle and some padded shorts – they'll make you feel a lot more comfortable.
- Invest in a water bottle that fits on to your bike, as it's easy to get dehydrated if you go out cycling for longer periods.

WEIGHT-TRAINING

Weight-training is an ultra-effective way to strengthen your muscles from top-to-toe. It'll also give you the brilliant body confidence that comes when you feel strong and toned.

How will it help my running?

By building strong, toned muscles you'll get faster and reduce your risk of injury. Weight-training is also great if you're trying to lose weight — the more muscle you gain, the more calories you'll burn. As the excess weight comes off, you'll find that each and every run starts to feel easier and more enjoyable.

What type of weights are best?

Free weights (such as hand-weights or dumbbells) will encourage you to use your whole body, and will get you working harder than using fixed weights machines at the gym. If you're a total beginner, you ideally need to start with a general weight-training programme for four to six weeks, which works all the major muscle groups of the body to get you ready for lifting heavier weights. Ask a trainer to put together a programme for you, or try a weights class at a gym. If that goes well, you can then move up to lifting heavier weights (see below).

How often do I need to do it?

Once you're lifting heavier weights, you'll need to do two sessions a week to get results. Again, ask a trainer to put together a programme of key moves for you. Aim to do 6–8 repetitions (reps) of each move, and to repeat each set of repetitions 6–8 times, with a 2-minute rest between sets. The idea is to lift weights that are heavy enough that by the last of the reps in each set, you feel you can't do any more.

Any top tips?

- This is one area where it's really, really worth going to a class, or having a personal training session, to learn how to do the exercises correctly. Get your technique right as soon as you start so you don't develop bad habits and injure yourself later on.

- Don't be afraid of weights. Lots of women shy away from them because they are scared of 'bulking up,' but really, you won't! What you will gain is better posture, body confidence and body shape.
- To develop strong legs, do squats and lunges holding dumbbells by your sides, or a barbell across your shoulders.

YOGA AND PILATES

Going to a regular yoga or Pilates class makes you stronger and more flexible, and teaches you great body awareness. Over time you'll learn to think of your body as one whole entity that works together, rather than a series of non-connected body parts.

How will they help my running?

Both yoga and Pilates will boost your strength and work on your flexibility. Pilates has a particular focus on strengthening your abdominal muscles and back, which will help you maintain good posture when you run, and may also help make you less injury prone. Both will teach you to stretch safely, again helping to reduce the risk of injury.

Which types of yoga and Pilates are best?

All kinds will bring you benefits, so choose the type that you like best. Some yoga teachers focus a lot on breathing, others teach dynamic forms of yoga such as Ashtanga, and others take Bikram classes which are performed in heated rooms to really make you sweat and help you improve

your flexibility. When it comes to Pilates, you can do mat-based Pilates, or use special equipment to work out on. See what's available in your area, and if you don't like one class, or your instructor's teaching style, don't be afraid to swap until you find something you're more comfortable with.

How often do I need to do them?

Aim to go to a class each week, and once you're familiar with some of the moves, you can use those you find most helpful on a daily basis, perhaps before or after runs to help prepare or relax you.

ANY TOP TIPS?

- Leave your competitive instincts at home – these classes aren't about trying to get into a more advanced position than your neighbour; they're about focusing on how your body feels, and calming your mind.
- Don't push yourself too hard too soon. You might not feel as if you're doing much in your first session, but it's deceptive, and you'll really feel it the next day.
- Use the body awareness you gain in classes to really tune into how your body feels – and where you might be storing stress – while you're out on a run.

YOUR HALF-MARATHON PLAN

WHO'S IT GOOD FOR?
Aspiring marathon runners who want to gauge how far they can go.

- **How does it feel?** Pretty special. Complete a half-marathon and you've already done more than most people ever will.

- **How long will it take?** Under 1:45 and you're a speed demon; about 2:00 is respectable; heading for 2:30 and you're towards the back (but that's where the interesting people are!)

- **What's the plan?** It's a 12-weeker designed by BUPA sports scientist Andy Ellis. If you're worried about tackling this distance, take a peek at our walk/run advice on page 162.

Don't forget to warm up before each session (see pages 116–117) and cool down and stretch (see pages 118–119) afterwards.

WEEK 1
Monday: Rest
Tuesday: Run 30 mins (effort level 5)
Wednesday: Run 30 mins (effort level 5)
Thursday: Rest
Friday: Run 30 mins (effort level 5)
Saturday: Rest
Sunday: Run 35 mins (effort level 6) – about 5K (3 miles)!

WEEK 2
Monday: Rest
Tuesday: Run 30 mins (effort level 5)
Wednesday: Run 30 mins (effort level 6–7), or test yourself with a 30-min tempo session (see overleaf)

Thursday: Rest
Friday: Run 30 mins (effort level 5)
Saturday: Rest
Sunday: Run 45 mins (effort level 6)

WEEK 3
Monday: Rest
Tuesday: Run 30 mins (effort level 5)
Wednesday: Run 40 mins (effort level 6–7), or try a 40-min tempo session (see overleaf)
Thursday: Rest
Friday: Run 30 mins (effort level 5)
Saturday: Rest
Sunday: Run 55 mins (effort level 6) – about 8K (5 miles)!

WEEK 4
Monday: Rest
Tuesday: Run 40 mins (effort level 5)
Wednesday: Run 50 mins (effort level 6–7), or do a 50-min tempo session (see overleaf)
Thursday: Rest
Friday: Run 30 mins (effort level 5), or if you're feeling lively, try 28 mins of intervals (see overleaf)
Saturday: Rest
Sunday: Run 65 mins (effort level 6)

WEEK 5
Monday: Rest
Tuesday: Run 40 mins (effort level 5)
Wednesday: Run 30 mins (effort level 6–7), or do a 30-min tempo session (see overleaf)
Thursday: Rest
Friday: Run 40 mins (effort level 5), or try 28 mins of intervals (see overleaf)
Saturday: Rest
Sunday: Run 80 mins (effort level 6)

WEEK 6
Monday: Rest
Tuesday: Run 40 mins (effort level 5)
Wednesday: Run 50 mins (effort level 6–7), or do a 50-min tempo session (see overleaf)
Thursday: Rest
Friday: Run 30 mins (effort level 5), or do 34 mins of intervals (see overleaf)
Saturday: Rest
Sunday: Run 90 mins (effort level 6) – about 13K (8 miles)!

WEEK 7
Monday: Rest
Tuesday: Run 40 mins (effort level 5)
Wednesday: Run 40 mins (effort level 6–7), or do a 40-min tempo session (see overleaf)
Thursday: Rest
Friday: Run 40 mins (effort level 5) or do 34 mins of intervals (see overleaf)
Saturday: Rest
Sunday: Run 65 mins (effort level 6)

WEEK 8
Monday: Rest
Tuesday: Run 40 mins (effort level 5)
Wednesday: Run 40 mins (effort level 6–7), or do a 40-min tempo session (see overleaf)
Thursday: Rest
Friday: Run 40 mins (effort level 5) or do 25 mins of intervals (see overleaf)
Saturday: Rest
Sunday: Run 110 mins (effort level 6) – about 16K (10 miles)!

WEEK 9
Monday: Rest
Tuesday: Run 40 mins (effort level 5)
Wednesday: Run 50 mins (effort level 6–7), or do a 50-min tempo session

Thursday: Rest
Friday: Run 50 mins (effort level 5), or do 25 mins of intervals (see overleaf)
Saturday: Rest
Sunday: Run 55 mins (effort level 6)

WEEK 10
Monday: Rest
Tuesday: Run 40 mins (effort level 5)
Wednesday: Run 40 mins (effort level 6–7), or do a 40-min tempo session (see overleaf)
Thursday: Rest
Friday: Run 40 mins (effort level 5), or do 25 mins of intervals (see overleaf)
Saturday: Rest
Sunday: Run 120 mins (effort level 6) – about 16K to 19K (10–12 miles)!

WEEK 11
Monday: Rest
Tuesday: Run 40 mins (effort level 5)
Wednesday: Run 40 mins (effort level 6–7), or do a 40-min tempo session (see overleaf)
Thursday: Rest
Friday: Run 40 mins (effort level 5), or do any of the interval sessions (see overleaf)
Saturday: Rest
Sunday: Run 65 mins (effort level 6)

WEEK 12
Monday: Rest
Tuesday: Run 30 mins (effort level 5)
Wednesday: Run 40 mins (effort 6–7), or do a 40-min tempo session (see overleaf), optional
Thursday: Rest
Friday: Run 30 mins (effort level 5)
Saturday: Rest
Sunday: HALF-MARATHON! (effort level 5–6)

MARATHON MAGIC

JUST ABOUT EVERYONE WHO HAS RUN A MARATHON AGREES IT'S A DAY IN A MILLION. WE QUIZZED SOME PROUD FINISHERS ABOUT TAKING ON THE ULTIMATE CHALLENGE …

'Running the London Marathon with my husband was certainly an experience – we went through every emotion in those 4½ hours, from quiet tension at the start line, laughing and joking at how clever we were when we passed the halfway mark, a huge row at 30K (19 miles) over our pace (when we decided it was probably best not to talk for a few miles), to **holding hands and literally falling into each other's arms as we crossed the finish line.** It was such an amazing feeling. The crowd support is unbelievable, it's like getting a little shot of adrenaline. After weeks of really tough training when I thought about giving up nearly every day, I had one of the best and most memorable days of my life.'
Rebecca Frank, 29, journalist, Bath

'I'd always trained for the New York City Marathon listening to music on my Walkman, and I found that really fast dance music helped me keep to a pace. So when I went over to America to run the marathon all on my own, I asked two friends to make me a tape of songs to listen to during the race, and asked them to speak on it and cheer me on. They chose things I'd never have thought of – like 'Reach For The Stars' by S Club 7 – which kept surprising me, and **they even said things like, "Come on, Rach, you can do it" between songs, which was just like having pats on the back all the way round.** When I finished the race, I wanted the whole of New York to lift me on their shoulders because it was such an achievement for me!'
Rachel Armitage, 29, charity worker, Sheffield

'A route that takes you through herds of zebra and acacia groves must make the Lewa Downs Marathon in Kenya one of the most remarkable races in the world. Sunrise finds herds of elephant and rhinoceros along the roadside and prides of lions asleep on the track. The race begins early, with helicopters, spotter planes and rangers fanning out in the pre-dawn light to make sure any dangerous wildlife has moved away from the roads. **Game rangers keep a watchful eye on proceedings as the runners, walkers and strollers enjoy spectacular views of Mount Kenya** – as well as herds of game at the roadside. I cannot think of any better way to appreciate the natural beauty of the African savannah grasslands.'
Mukesh Kerai, 32, systems engineer, Sydney, Australia

'They say that getting married or having kids are two landmark events in your life. To me, running a marathon is up there with both. My first marathon, the Brighton Marathon in April 2011, was the second most incredible day of my life (the first being my wedding day). The atmosphere on race day was electric, the support from the locals was amazing and I didn't hit the wall because I'd fuelled up so well (which really means I'd scoffed plenty of food beforehand!). **When I queued up at the start, I could hardly believe I was about to tackle 26.2 miles, yet I felt calm and strangely confident, probably because I'd done so much training.** I knew how much completing the distance meant to me, so I knew I'd finish no matter what. I didn't break any amazing time barriers, but it was utterly exhilarating crossing that finish line. Running a marathon should be on everyone's bucket list. The sense of achievement you feel afterwards is second to none.'
Christina Macdonald, 45, editor-in-chief, *Women's Running* UK

'I decided to run the London Marathon as a personal challenge. It was something I'd watched friends do and never dreamed I'd manage myself, but I built up by doing short races and realized I could do it. I was never fast – my goal was just to run the whole way, and I did – even though sometimes I was at a snail's pace! On the start line I felt terrified, but as the gun went off, all my panic melted away. **Running along, I had such an amazing, sociable time, singing and chatting to people.** I had a wobble around 17 miles, but some friends who were watching ran alongside me and got me back on track, and from then on, I knew I'd make it. Running for the finish line, the tune to *Chariots of Fire* was playing in my head, and I wanted those moments to last forever. I finished in 5 hours, and floated around on a high for days. I'd astounded myself and my friends!'
Lindsay Cunningham, 34, teacher, Hampshire

'I ran the London Marathon four weeks after having an ovary removed. Standing on the start line, I couldn't believe I'd made it. **I ran with my sister Louise, and finished in just over 4½ hours with a few tears and big hugs along the way.** It was only a month after the race, when I'd come down off my high, that the impact of what I'd been through really hit me. I'm convinced that being so fit and healthy is what helped me recover so quickly from the operation, and having the marathon to focus on helped me through what could have been a really traumatic time.'
Rebecca Lake, 31, PA, York

MORE MARATHON MAGIC

'They say life begins at 40 – or at least my running career did! I live a stone's throw from the start of the London Marathon and every year I found myself completely choked up by this amazing event. The year I hit 40, I applied for a place, despite having only ever run for about 15 minutes at a time and being known as the Queen of the Black Cab! My first run outside was on New Year's Eve and I ached for Britain while everyone else celebrated. But things got better – I had chickenpox in my mid-30s and had tried everything to ease the post-viral fatigue that dogged me for years. Miraculously, running magicked away all the back and shoulder problems it had left me with. Thanks to my job, I even found myself swapping running tips with Alastair Campbell a few days before the London Marathon. And it really was one fantastically memorable day.'
Jackie Graveney, 41, PR executive, London

'I and a few running friends have been training disabled people to run for quite a few years. It has given us untold rewards and enjoyment to see them develop and go from despair to becoming pillars of their communities. I took my first blind runner through the 89K (55.6 mile) Comrades Marathon in South Africa in 1985, and he moaned for almost the entire 10½ hours as I pulled and tugged him up the hills. I kept him cool by pouring cups of cold water over his head every now and again. When I told him he was near the end of the race, he managed to get what he thought was a cup of water and promptly poured it over my head as a token of appreciation for what I'd been doing for him. Unfortunately, the cup he'd been handed was full of warm Coca-Cola! I was not at all happy with him, as you can imagine!'
Denis Tabakin, 62, footwear consultant, Johannesburg, South Africa

'If someone had told me a few years ago that I'd be lining up at the start of the 2002 London Marathon next to Paula Radcliffe, I would have laughed in their face. Since my first running experience had seen me struggling to make it twice round a field only a few years before, this scenario seemed extremely unlikely. But amazingly, even though I started running late in life, I improved really fast and was soon good enough to line up with the elite women! I can now run the sorts of times I initially would only have dreamed of (my marathon personal best is 3:01). I've gained so much from running – friends, a husband (I met him at the running club!), a leaner body, a much healthier attitude to life, and, of course, my five minutes of fame as I lined up in the London marathon next to Paula Radcliffe and waved to my mum!'
Pippa Major, 37, e-commerce development manager, Surrey

'What I love about doing a marathon is that the buzz and sense of achievement never go away. The memory of turning the corner of The Mall into the final straight of the London Marathon and seeing the clock with those big yellow digits ticking over is as vivid as the memory of when my daughter was born and laid on my chest. It sounds disproportionate, but the months of commitment involved make finishing a marathon a very special moment.'
Emma Simpson, 31, designer, London

'I'd already done a few marathons and triathlons, and so finally worked up the bottle to tackle the Ironman UK Triathlon. It starts with a 2.4 mile swim, then a 112 mile bike ride, and you finish by running a marathon. Amazingly I felt relatively OK when I got off the bike after 7½ hours of cycling, and started running – the sun was shining, and my sisters were playing the theme tune to Rocky on a little portable CD player as I set off!

   I ran the first 13 miles in about 2 hours, which I was delighted with, but by then I was running out of energy. I knew there was a photographer on the course so I kept going until I'd passed him as I didn't want to get snapped walking! But then, I ended up walking the next 10 miles. By now we'd been on the go for over 11 hours and it was totally dark. But, finally, with 2 miles to go, I started running again. I wanted to do it in under 15 hours, and even managed to put in a sprint at the end, finishing in 14:49. I celebrated by swapping Lucozade for lager. Although the training took over my life for a while, I do think I'd like to do another one as I really enjoyed feeling that fit. Next time, I'd be aiming to finish in under 14 hours, though!'
James Danaher, 32, lawyer, London

'It's weird, but for some reason I can't recall any of the bad bits of the Edinburgh Marathon, only the good ones. Whereas I find it really hard to remember how battered my legs and knees felt, the memories that never seem to fade are the haunting sound of bagpipes in the mist at the start, seeing the magnificent Forth Rail Bridge in the distance and the exhilaration as I crossed the finish line.'
Graham Williams, 50, intelligence analyst, London

'Runners frolicking about in fancy dress and glorious vineyard views - the Bacchus Marathon was a total hoot! It was held on Denbies Wine Estate in Dorking, Surrey, and my main aim was to sample all the fabulous wines on offer at the refreshment stops but still make it to the finish, where a hog roast (and more free wine) awaited. Thankfully the wine was served in tiny cups so I succeeded on both counts, even though the hilly course was surprisingly tough!'
Penny Mills, 26, teacher, Brighton

ONE MINUTE EVERYTHING'S GOING BRILLIANTLY AND YOU'RE ENJOYING YOUR RUNNING, AND THE NEXT MINUTE DISASTER STRIKES. MAYBE YOU'VE RUN OUT OF STEAM, HIT A MOTIVATION CRISIS, PICKED UP AN INJURY, OR SIMPLY STOPPED SEEING RESULTS? WELL, DON'T PANIC BECAUSE WE KNOW HOW TO PICK YOU UP AND SET YOU BACK ON YOUR FEET ...

9. GET OVER IT

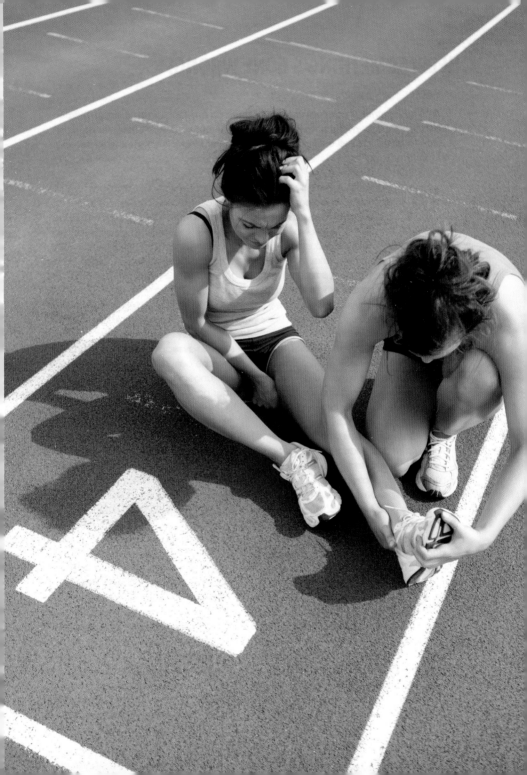

WANT TO HEAR SOMETHING AMAZING? THEN READ THE STORIES OF THESE NINE TRULY EXCEPTIONAL RUNNERS FROM AROUND THE WORLD WHO WERE SO DETERMINED TO RUN THAT THEY OVERCAME OBSTACLES THAT WOULD HAVE STOPPED MOST ORDINARY PEOPLE IN THEIR TRACKS. THEY'RE LIVING PROOF THAT WHERE THERE'S A WILL, THERE'S A WAY ...

10. GET AMAZED

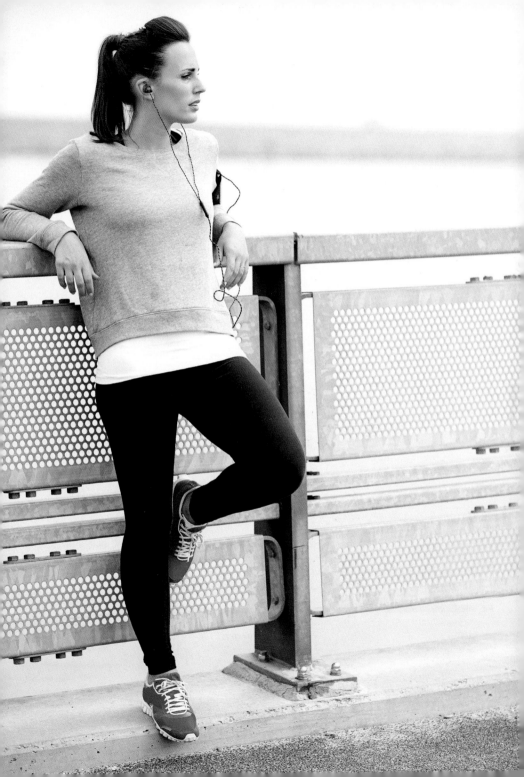

'RUNNING HELPED ME BEAT ALCOHOLISM'

While she was a teenager, VICTORIA BROCKHURST, 29, from London, battled addictions to alcohol and Valium, but now she faces entirely different challenges as she tackles some of the world's toughest ultra-marathons.

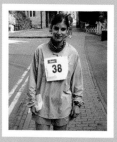

I started drinking at 13. I experimented with alcohol at a party, and from the very first time I tasted it, I drank until I passed out. I wasn't very happy at that time and alcohol made me feel more relaxed and extrovert. By the time I was 16, I was drinking two litres of vodka a day and my health had deteriorated dramatically. My liver was enlarged, I had a bleeding stomach ulcer and food made me feel sick. I smelled of alcohol even when I wasn't drinking because of the vodka I was sweating out. Things got so bad that, at the age of 17, I was asked to leave school and undergo a home detox supervised by my mum. I had to take Antabuse (a medication that makes you violently ill if you drink alcohol) and was prescribed Valium to help control the shaking and horrifying hallucinations that were the side effects of going cold turkey. I succeeded in giving up

drinking (though I developed an addiction to Valium) and four months later was allowed back at school to sit my exams. However, the day after my A-levels, I began drinking again.

The turning point came when, aged 19, I was admitted to A&E after I'd cut my finger while drinking. I heard the doctor telling a nurse I was 'a drunk' and that's when I said to myself, 'I don't want to do this any more.' A few days later, I checked into a rehab centre where I received treatment for my addictions.

When I came out of rehab, I knew I had to find something to replace the role alcohol had played in my life. I'd always been sporty, so I chose running. I didn't really enjoy my first session as my body was still very weak after everything it had been through in the detox. But I don't do things by halves, so I took to running in the way I had to drinking – I ran a lot! I decided to start racing, and over the next five years I went from doing 5Ks to completing the London Marathon.

I'd go for long runs, six days a week.

'I knew I had to find something to replace the role alcohol had played in my life and I chose running'

As an alcoholic, you're warned that when you stop drinking you might try to replace alcohol with something else. I knew I had the ability to go overboard with my running and so had to be careful not get too obsessed.

New life

I worked as a chef after leaving school but after getting so into running, I retrained as a personal trainer and now run a fitness company. I fundraise for Sport Against Addiction, which works with the charity Action On Addiction, to raise awareness of addiction, and I hope my story will help others beat their addictions, too.

A few years ago, I competed in the Marathon des Sables, a 243K (151 mile) race that takes place over six days in the Moroccan desert and is often billed as 'the world's toughest foot race'. An unexpected bonus was that it led to me meeting my future husband Dan while doing an 87K (54 mile) race in preparation for it.

He held a gate open for me along the route and when I saw him at the finish, we agreed to pair up for a few more training sessions. Six weeks later, we did the Marathon des Sables together in scorching temperatures that often reached 40°C. We were elated to finish, particularly as my dad was waiting at the finish line – and five months later Dan and I got engaged!

The Marathon of Britain was our next challenge. It involved running 282K (175 miles) over six days. The weather was really hot, and the hilly course meant it felt even tougher than the Marathon des Sables. Then came the Trans 333 in Egypt, a 360K (224 mile) race when I ran virtually non-stop for about three days. I was too afraid to sleep because every time I lay down and shut my eyes, I was worried that I wouldn't be able to start running again! It was scary, but exhilarating, being on my own in the desert.

I'm just so thankful for what running's done for me. It's helped me stay sober for ten years by giving me new goals to aim for, and has also given me belief in myself. I used to drink when I was sad or depressed, but now I go running. Everything always seems better after a run. In fact, you could say that running has taught me to be happy!

HOW VICTORIA DID IT

Motivation tip: 'Join a club or run with a running partner – it'll help you push yourself harder and having an appointment means you're less likely not to go.'

Training tip: 'It's OK to walk! Don't give yourself a hard time about it if you have to – just remind yourself that it's better to walk than to stop!'

'I LOST OVER HALF MY BODYWEIGHT'

Weighing 121kg (19st 1lb), JULIE PRINCE, 37, from Reading couldn't even climb the stairs without getting out of breath. Now she's an incredible 62kg (9st 11lb) lighter – all thanks to running.

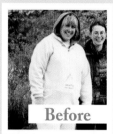

Before

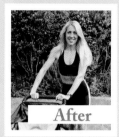

After

At my biggest, I was a size 24 and weighed 121kg (19st 1lb). I got dizzy just walking up stairs, and thought I'd never, ever be able to run. Just 18 months later, having taken up running and changed my eating habits, I'd lost 62kg (9st 11lb) and slimmed down to a size 10! The change in my body and my health is unbelievable – I'm half my previous size and I've found I'm actually good at something I never thought I could do in a million years.

I was first put on a diet aged ten by my GP, and by secondary school I was a size 16 and one of the biggest girls in my class. I slimmed down to 76kg (12st) for my wedding day but soon piled the weight back on again. Things got worse when my husband's job moved us to Aberdeen in Scotland. Feeling isolated, lonely and bored, I took refuge in comfort eating.

I found a new job as a teacher but the pupils ridiculed me about my size and one nicknamed me 'Titanic'. I was still reasonably confident as my husband never criticized my weight and complimented me on other things like my hair and nails. However, my size really hit home when I couldn't do up a size 22 blazer I'd bought for an interview and could barely get a bath towel to meet round my body. I remember crying because I couldn't find anything to wear to a party, and my husband making me a dress himself to try to help me feel better.

I finally started losing weight in an attempt to shape up for a friend's wedding, having got the shock of my life after standing on the scales and watching them tip to 121kg (19st 1lb). I'm quite tall – 1.73m (5ft 8in) – but I realized half of me had to go! I didn't begin running straightaway – instead, I started very gently with swimming and walking, and just eating healthy meals rather than following a diet. It took me nine months to lose the first 32kg (5st), and it was at this stage that I discovered running.

My husband's job had taken us to Tunisia, and we were living in a village in a compound with security guards and a 750m (½ mile) track that ran right round it. One of our friends bet me that I couldn't even make it round the track once. I set off on my own to prove him wrong, and ran six laps, very slowly, stopping between each one. Inspired, my husband and I decided to join the group of Brits in our village who were training to do their first half-marathon.

'I began to slim down and when I fitted into a pair of size 20 jeans thought I was the cat's whiskers'

Tricks and tactics

The first few runs were really hard. Although I wasn't the biggest in the group, I was at the back, and I hated feeling so breathless and under pressure to keep up. We combined jogging and walking, going round and round the track, often late at night because of the heat. To help me stay motivated, I used a workbook that I'd take everywhere with me. I wrote down every run I did, everything I ate, every compliment anyone paid me, and the date when I got out of the seriously overweight bracket of the weight chart. I even drew a weight-loss graph to keep me on track. Once I started running, the line on the graph began to plummet, and I went from losing 0.25kg (½lb) a week to losing just over 1kg (2½lb) a week. It was an amazing motivator to have found something that had such an effect on my body.

Although at the start losing 19kg (3st) didn't feel as if it made a huge difference because I had so very far to go, by now I was noticing significant changes. My stomach was slimming down and I remember how overjoyed I felt when I fitted into a pair of size 20 white jeans – I thought I was the cat's whiskers!

I ran my first race about five months later when I came back to England for a summer holiday, and it felt like a big milestone. I was very, very nervous and unwittingly had chosen a really fast 10K (6 mile) race that was full of good club runners. I'd made my way to the very front as I thought I'd need a bit of a head start, and ended up getting elbowed by all the fast runners trying to get by! Running towards the finish line, I heard one of the marshals say I was last, so I put on a spurt and beat the two other ladies in front of me to come in third from last. Although I'd not exactly picked an ideal first race to try, I was on a real high about my time – a very respectable 56 minutes – and felt very proud of myself.

Next came the half-marathon I'd trained for with the group. It took place in Florence, Italy. I'd reached my goal weight (63.6kg/10st) and was feeling brilliant. I already knew I was going to make the distance as I'd run 30 laps of our track in the compound – the equivalent of a half-marathon. But I was desperate to get round in under 2 hours, which I did, and achieving that goal set me off wanting to try to run the London Marathon in under 4 hours.

Something else that made the half-marathon feel very special was that just afterwards we found out I was expecting our daughter Helena – I'd run the race without even realizing it! I kept on running gently throughout my pregnancy and afterwards I lost 6.4kg (1st) more than my pre-pregnancy weight, partly because I was breastfeeding, and partly because I was training for the marathon.

Perfect day
By now, we'd moved back to England, and I would set off with Helena in her running buggy, run the 6.5K (4 miles) into town, have my treat, which was a latte, then run home again. I loved the variety of being able to run to visit other places rather than having just to run round in circles in the compound. I also used the running as thinking and planning time.

I stuck to my training religiously for the marathon, and consequently everything went right for me on the day and I finished in 3 hours and 51 minutes. It was truly brilliant, and even now, thinking about the day and the atmosphere sends tingles down my spine.

Running has been great in other ways, too. I'm confident enough to go

running in shorts and a crop top, and I can buy size 10 clothes off the rail and wear whatever I want because my weight has now stabilized at 59kg (9st 4lb). It's also done so much for my health and I have lots more energy.

Slow but sure
Now I'm keen to run another marathon soon, but recently I've also been helping some of my friends to start running, explaining to them how important it is to start off slowly. I firmly believe that being patient is the key to both learning to run and losing weight. Lots of people want a fast solution, and the more weight they have to lose, the quicker they want to lose it. But if you learn to go slow, you can achieve anything – I'm living proof!

HOW JULIE DID IT
Motivation tip: 'Keep a record of the progress you make – I wrote absolutely everything down. I even devised a sticker system, awarding myself a gold star every time I completed an exercise session.'
Diet tip: 'I try to copy the way my husband eats, to keep me relaxed about food and stop me falling back into the "I'm a big person trying to lose weight" mentality. If he wants a biscuit, he goes ahead and has one, and so do I.'

'RUNNING HAS BEEN MY SAVIOUR'

Having suffered years of severe depression, BERYL THOMAS, 52, became a virtual prisoner in her own home. Now a keen runner, she's fully recovered, 28.6kg (4st 7lb) lighter and pounding the streets of Darwen, England, wearing angel wings and an ear-to-ear grin.

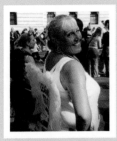

I'd always been a really bouncy, happy-go-lucky person, but about ten years ago I became severely depressed. It was partly due to money worries, and I'd also taken on too much in my job as a childminder. I had to give up work, and I'd sit at home rocking and staring into space, unable to stop crying. I tried everything from Prozac to electric shock therapy, but nothing seemed to work, and eventually things became so bad that I even tried to take an overdose. I became incredibly withdrawn, and if someone knocked on my front door, I'd get down on my hands and knees and hide behind the sofa rather than answer it.

It was a terrible time, not just for me, but also for my husband, Howard, my twin daughters, Katie and Kelly, now 22, and my son, Anthony, now 17, who had to go through the trauma of seeing me so ill. It got so bad that I couldn't leave the house, and the only time I'd go out was to go food shopping with Howard. I was like a frightened child, clinging to his arm and having panic attacks. After almost ten years of battling against depression, things finally changed for me in May 2001. It was getting light very early in the morning and, although I can't quite explain why, I suddenly felt I wanted to get out of the house. I got up at 5.30am and went for a walk on the edge of the moors where I knew no one would be about, never giving my safety a second thought. Although going out alone felt very frightening, the sense of freedom I experienced being away from those four walls was amazing. I realized from day one that getting outside and getting moving gave me a high.

After I'd been out a few times, I started to think I could try to run a few steps. At first, I could manage only ten steps before my chest felt as if it was going to explode. My medication and comfort eating had made my weight soar to 95.5kg (15st) and I was wearing a dress size 22, so I found running terribly hard and got very red in the face. But I saw it as a challenge and began counting how many steps I could manage, aiming to run for 100 steps. The first time that I could run all the way back to my house, I was literally jumping for joy.

I also started going to meetings at Weight Watchers, taking my daughter Kelly along for moral support, but I was very nervous and sat right at the back of the class not wanting to be noticed or say anything. It was a slow process, but the running helped my confidence grow day by day, and by July, I'd plucked up the courage to enter a race – the Great Women's Run in

'The first time that I could run all the way back to my house, I was literally jumping for joy'

Manchester. It's a wonderful race that gives you the chance to run down Coronation Street where the soap opera is filmed. Although it was only 8K (5 miles), it took me well over two hours to finish.

After a while, the combination of dieting and exercising began to work and I got slimmer all over. I started losing a couple of pounds each week and found that even my neck and feet changed shape! The more weight I lost, the more confident, happy and in control I felt, and I even managed to go back to work.

One day close to Christmas, I was in town shopping and I saw some angel wings in a shop. I don't know what hit me, but I just thought I'd stick them on my back when I was out running for a bit of a laugh. My son Anthony was horrified and said I wasn't to go out in them, and to be honest I felt pretty silly the first time I wore them. My heart was really pounding as I put them on, and I even wore sunglasses and a cap so no one would be able to recognize me! The reaction I got was amazing, as by this time I was running all over town and

on busy roads. Drivers would toot their horns at me and workmen couldn't believe their eyes. My daughter Kelly made little signs for me on the computer to wear on my back – one said 'Angel In Training' and another said 'Looking For Heaven'. The more I ran, the more daring I became. I collected a whole selection of wings – ones with feathers, diamanté and lace. Even the local radio station spotted me and ran a competition to find out who I was. When it tracked me down, they interviewed me on air about what I was up to. I was amazed at the way the whole thing had snowballed, and just had to explain I was wearing them for fun. Even so, I earned the nickname 'The Angel of the North', after the huge statue of an angel that stands on a hillside outside Newcastle upon Tyne.

In 2002 I ran the Great Women's Run in Manchester again, this time with my wings on. My daughter Katie was even inspired to run the race with me, though she'd never run before. By this time, I'd lost about 28.6kg (4st 7lb) and was feeling great. I got a place right at the front with all the elite runners and set off with them with a really serious look on my face (wearing my wings!) because I wanted to do a really good time.

Guardian angel

Soon after the race, I finally came off my medication and decided I wanted to do the London Marathon the following year. I was determined to do it as a celebration of my twin daughters' 21st birthday, and to raise money for the neonatal department that had looked after them when they'd been born prematurely. The day I found out I'd got a place in the marathon through the ballot, I was literally whooping for joy. I did all of my training with my angel wings on – by then, they had just become a part of me. They were really appropriate, too, as I'd become convinced that I had a guardian angel watching over me, keeping me safe and motivated.

Learning to fly

On marathon day all my nerves had gone and I was on a complete high, wearing my wings with feathers on and a sign saying 'Learning To Fly'. Although I found it hard and got very tired and dehydrated, somehow I found the will to keep going. The crowds were brilliant. I hadn't known you were meant to write your name on your T-shirt so people could shout for you, but it didn't matter – they all just shouted, 'Go on Angel!' All

I could do was cry, and not quietly – I was really wailing! When I saw the finish line, it was like Christmas and birthdays all rolled into one. I crossed the line beaming for all the photographs!

Leading the way

Running really has been my saviour. Looking back, I can't believe how poorly I'd been and how much running turned things round for me. My husband teases me that I've now got a bony bottom, and I can even fit into my daughters' clothes! I've turned into a kind of running Pied Piper – other women ask if they can run with me and turn to me for advice. I'm happy to help them because I'm just so grateful to be back to my old happy self again. Even now, I still say a little thank you to my guardian angel before and after every run.

HOW BERYL DID IT

Motivation tip: 'I have little motivational things I repeat to myself in my head, such as 'Keep focused' and 'When you've got the ball, you've got to run with it.' They help stop me running out of steam when I'm finding it hard.'

Eating tip: 'Take one day of eating at a time. Don't worry about what you ate yesterday or what you're going to eat tomorrow, just concentrate on getting today right.'

'AFTER HAVING CANCER I APPRECIATE EVERY RUN'

After undergoing chemotherapy for testicular cancer at the age of 18, ANDREW SHIPPEY, from Leeds, was unable even to walk. But running got him back on his feet – and enabled him to raise an astounding half a million pounds for research into fighting cancer.

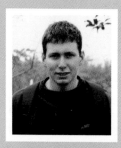

Seven years ago, testicular cancer tore a big hole in my life. I was just your average 18-year-old when I was diagnosed and told I had a 50/50 chance of survival. But I did survive, and four years later I triumphantly finished the Great North Run half-marathon, feeling absolutely amazing.

Most people watching the race that day wouldn't have guessed how hard I had to fight to get there, and that I had tens of thousands of people supporting me and resting their hopes on me. And even I didn't know that by crossing that finish line, I'd raised more than £500,000 to fund research into the disease that nearly killed me. Through running I regained my fitness and transformed a terrible situation into a life-affirming one.

Shocked and devastated

Before I developed cancer, I was very active – I was a regular runner and loved football. It was while I was playing football during the Easter break at university that I first realized I was ill. I remember the date exactly: Tuesday, 8 April. I got a knock in the stomach and felt so sick that I threw up. In A&E, the doctors suspected I had a burst ulcer, but they conducted further tests just to be sure. Things moved at lightning speed after that: on 10 April I was told I had cancer. Two days later, I was having chemotherapy.

The doctors waited for my mum and dad to arrive before they told me the bad news. I was devastated and shocked but felt I had to put on a brave face in front of them. Once they'd gone home, I kept thinking, 'You're 18 and you're dying,' and kept asking, 'Why me?' But I woke up the next day with a completely different attitude. There was no way I was going to let cancer beat me, and I had an unshakeable conviction that I was going to get better. I kept telling myself that testicular cancer is 95% curable if it's caught early.

However, after my first chemo session, I was dealt another blow when I was told the cancer had spread to my liver and lungs and there was now only a 50/50 chance I'd survive. My dad was nearly in tears but I just laughed it off as I was 100% certain I was going to get better. The doctors suggested a high-dose chemotherapy that was so toxic they'd have to harvest stem cells from my blood to help replace all the healthy cells it would kill along with the cancerous ones.

The chemotherapy knocked me for six. I was hospitalized for five weeks, spent four days in intensive care and was so ill that I don't remember two weeks of that time. Afterwards, I had to

'There was no way I was going to let cancer beat me – I had an unshakeable conviction I was going to get better'

have hours of physio to help me walk again as I'd been flat on my back for so long. I also had to have two operations.

Joy and relief

I'll never forget the day I got the all-clear in October. I'd gone for a check-up after my operation and expected to be told I'd need one more dose of chemotherapy but the doctor told me it wouldn't be necessary. I wanted to jump up and kiss her! My mum was with me and when we got outside I said, 'I told you I could do it!' I spent the rest of the day visiting my friends to tell them the good news before hitting the pub. I can't begin to describe the sore head I had the next day – but I didn't care!

Starting over

I was determined from then on to get the most out of life every single day. As a first step, I set my sights on playing in a singles-versus-marrieds football match my club had organized, and started running to get fit for it. On my first run I got so carried away that I went way too far too soon and ended up aching

like hell for several days afterwards. However, it felt great being able to do something I wanted to do for a change instead of having my whole life dictated to me as it had been when I was in hospital.

I made it through the match and the following year I went back to university to complete my degree. I continued running and the following year decided to do the Great North Run in Newcastle upon Tyne. I thought I'd gain an enormous sense of achievement doing something like that: to beat cancer you have to be tough, which is exactly what you have to be to run 21K (13.1 miles). I found the race quite challenging, but then so did the friends I ran with. I had no difficulty keeping up with them and didn't seem to have been affected by my illness. That year and the next, I raised about £100 each time for Cancer Research UK and was really chuffed with that.

Payback time

Then came a call from Cancer Research UK who said it was looking for someone to run the Great North

Run, around whom it could base a big charity fundraising campaign. I readily agreed as I was really keen to give something back to them. I knew I owed my life to it – the high-dose chemo I'd been given had been developed with the help of one of its grants.

I had an awesome time on the day – the atmosphere at the start, when we lined up with a crowd of more than 30,000 people, was amazing. I ran with eight friends and we stuck together throughout, chatting, laughing and encouraging each other. It was much hotter than it had been in previous years and I was near to collapse not far from the end when a kind person in the crowd handed me a biscuit that gave me a huge sugar – and morale – boost. I knew I simply had to make it to the finish line as I had so much money riding on me – an astonishing £370,000! When I finally got to the end, I thought, 'The money's in the bank!'

Amazing support
But the best was yet to come. Several weeks later, Cancer Research UK called to say that a mailshot it had sent out after the race had raised even more sponsorship and that my total was now a staggering £533,000. I was speechless and very touched that more than 32,000 people had sponsored me, including a pensioner who'd called Cancer Research UK to ask what my race number was. She said she and her friends in the old people's home wanted to be able to spot 'their boy' on the TV.

Hope and glory
I think the reason people responded to my appeal was that it was a good hope story – perhaps they thought, 'He's a young kid, he's had cancer, and yet he's willing to run 13 miles. He got off his backside to do something amazing.' I think I helped them see that there's life after cancer.

I've been clear of cancer for more than six years now, and will carry on doing the Great North Run for charity every year. I owe a lot to running – being fit before I became ill played a major role in my recovery. Running helped me build myself up again. Now, every time I go for a run I'm celebrating being alive.

HOW ANDREW DID IT
Motivation tip: 'Raise money for charity but choose something you care passionately about so you'll feel you're letting people down if you don't finish the race.'

Training tip: 'Always build up gradually and don't drain your body by overdoing it. And don't forget to ease up on your training the week before a race.'

'I RAN THE LONDON MARATHON – WHILE IN PRISON'

When FAY JOHNSON, 41, from London, went to prison for fraud, her self-esteem hit an all-time low. But being offered the chance to run the London Marathon while serving her sentence rebuilt her faith in herself and her abilities.

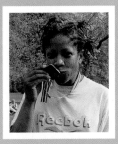

When I was sent to prison at HMP Downview, in Surrey, I found it incredibly hard to cope because everything was so different from the outside world. I had to leave behind my old life with my 14-year-old son and my partner, and face a four-year sentence inside. I started out in a tiny cell, with a toilet just a foot away from my bed and bars on the windows. Our doors were locked from 8pm until 8am, and the only thing I could do was sit in my cell and read my Bible. I didn't find it easy to get along with lots of the other prisoners and, although my faith helped me keep going, it was a truly terrible time.

We were allowed out of our cells during the day, so I started spending all my time at the prison gym. At 89kg (14st) and a size 18, I was incredibly unconfident, so I'd just sit on the exercise bike and pedal for hours. The PE officers noticed that I was going to the gym a lot and one, Linda Charles (whom everyone calls Charlie), offered me the chance to do a Community Sports Leader qualification, which I passed without any problem. All the exercise I had to do on the course also meant I slimmed down to about 67kg (10st 6lb). After that, Charlie offered me a job as a gym orderly and I was also moved into a nicer wing at the prison.

In early January one year the governor of the prison offered me a place in that year's London Marathon, raising money for a charity called The Hardman Trust, which helps rehabilitate prisoners. My first thought was, 'You've asked the wrong person, I can't possibly do it.' I'd never been a runner, and didn't think I could even run to the end of the road. But Charlie stepped in and reminded me that I didn't have to win, just finish. She told me she was convinced I could do it, which made me feel it would be an insult to her judgement to tell her I couldn't. Thinking about it alone in my cell, I realized it was the first time in ages that something nice had happened to me, so I plucked up the courage to say yes.

Shaky start

My first run was only a couple of minutes on the prison treadmill. My legs couldn't keep up with the pace of the machine, even when it was going really slowly, but Charlie just told me she believed in me and said I had to get on with it. From then on, I started running almost every day, and after ten days I was ecstatic when I ran a whole mile without stopping. It never felt easy, though, because as soon as I improved, Charlie moved the goalposts again to make things harder. Nevertheless, I started looking forward

> ## 'Three prison officers took it in turns to run on the treadmill beside me to help keep me motivated'

to my runs and enjoying the company I had while I was running – Charlie organized prison officers to take it in turns to run on the treadmill beside me to keep me motivated. The first time I ran 14.4K (9 miles), three officers each did 5K (3 mile) stints on the treadmill next to mine.

Mind games

After that, I was allowed outside to start running round the prison's Astroturf football pitch. By the end of February, I managed the magic total of 21K (13.1 miles) – a half-marathon – by running 93 laps. It was quite a challenge running round and round in circles, and to help me keep count of the laps I'd think about counting objects – like two apples to remind me I was on lap two – and so on. Running became like an escape for me, and despite being in prison, I felt a sense of freedom at being able to go off into my own thoughts. Even though I was feeling fitter, I still found it difficult to believe the marathon was really going to happen – it seemed like part of the outside world that I didn't live in any more.

Running free

Eight weeks before the marathon, I was allowed out of prison so Charlie could take me to buy trainers for the race. She had to get a special licence for the outing, but although she had to stay close by me, she didn't have to handcuff me. It was a real treat to see all the shops again. I wanted to go window shopping, but of course Charlie wouldn't let me!

After that, Charlie also applied to be able to take me running outside the prison. It felt very different running on the hard concrete instead of a soft treadmill or Astroturf, but it was wonderful to see things such as houses and gardens, which I hadn't seen for such a long time. Charlie also asked the prison kitchen to prepare pasta dishes for me and ordered bananas and sports drinks specially for me. All the other inmates and prison officers were very supportive of me as well.

The night before the marathon, I lay in my cell and thought about how proud I was that Charlie and the rest of the prison had put their trust in me, and how I didn't want to let them down. I also knew that a huge amount of my self-esteem rested on my getting round the marathon course.

The big day

On the morning of the marathon, I got up at 3am because I was so afraid of oversleeping. I had a big breakfast and set off really early with Charlie, heading for the start in Greenwich. Standing on the start line, I felt a lot more excited and nervous than I'd expected. I was allowed to run on my own, and just meet Charlie at the finish line. Rather than chatting to people, I kept my head down and tried to stay focused, but I really loved seeing all the London sights again, and also the way all the children in the crowd put their hands up to clap my hand as I ran by. I saw Charlie, who kept popping up at different points, and also met up with my partner and son at the finish line. I was surprised that even though it had taken me more than six hours to run the race, there were still huge crowds cheering us on, and I know my son was totally amazed to see me do something so sporty! I amazed myself, too, and now that it's all over, I still can't quite believe did it. I think if I didn't have my medal to prove it, it would feel like a dream.

Future hopes

What the marathon taught me is that if someone believes in you enough to offer a helping hand, you can achieve the unthinkable. I'm up for parole soon and can finally see a future for myself outside prison. Thanks to the running and the fitness course I did, I now have the confidence and ambition to set up my own fitness business, working with obese children.

As a thank you, I want to donate my marathon medal to Charlie as she put in as much hard work as I did! I know she was incredibly proud because she's never trained someone to run a marathon before. It's also a way of thanking her for trusting me, and giving me a chance to prove that I could do it. I would love it to hang in the prison gym and inspire other prisoners to do a marathon. I hope I've paved the way for them to have a go, too – and that they get just as much out of it as I did.

HOW FAY DID IT

Motivation tip: 'I only ever thought of my short-term goals. If Charlie set me a task, I always achieved it as I never wanted to come back and admit I couldn't do it.'

Eating tip: 'I started eating porridge for breakfast when I began training for the marathon, and I still have it now. It's really filling and satisfying but also low in calories.'

'NO ONE KNEW WHETHER I'D SURVIVE MY FALL'

A terrible accident left EMMA DOBINSON, 30, from London, in a coma and with a serious brain injury.
Now, four years on, she's made an amazing recovery, using running, and one special race, as her lifeline.

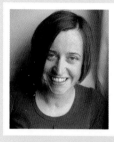

Before I had my accident, I was really sporty, and used to run regularly. Now, four years down the line, running has helped me claw my way back to feeling fit and healthy again. It took a lot of courage for me to dare to try running after what I'd been through, but I'm so glad I did because it really helped me recover both physically and emotionally.

The accident happened at about 1.30am one Monday morning. I was returning home in a taxi after a night out with friends, when I'd drunk far too much. I was also feeling absolutely shattered because I'd been really busy at work. The taxi driver said later that when he dropped me off, I didn't go into my house but set off down the road. I have no idea where I was going or why – in fact, I don't know anything about the lead-up to the accident except what I've since been told, because it wiped out part of my memory. I ended up at a block of nearby flats, where I fell about 4.5m (15ft) over the edge of the first-floor walkway. About four hours later, a stranger found me lying on the ground, bleeding heavily with a huge gash in my head and a mangled left arm.

Fighting for survival

I stayed in a coma for nearly two weeks. I had seriously injured my brain and the doctors had to remove a part of my skull to help reduce the pressure that had built up. They also had to insert long metal screws into my arm to repair my shattered elbow. When I first came round, I couldn't speak, and people had to interpret what I wanted from the expressions in my eyes and blinking alone. The whole thing was very traumatic for everyone – the police opened an investigation to try to find out whether anyone else had been involved or tried to hurt me, and also questioned me over whether I might have been trying deliberately to harm myself. They decided no one else was involved, but I still have to live with the uncertainty of not knowing exactly what happened or why.

My short-term memory was very badly affected by the fall and, once I started talking again, I'd get my words jumbled up (I'd tell my visitors to sit on the toilet, when I was pointing at a chair). I was also totally exhausted and had to spend hours sleeping. After four months in hospital, I was finally allowed to go back home, and that's when exercise started to play a role in my recovery. Having to cope with the outside world, and even silly things such as reading bank statements, felt like a lot to handle, and I was very upset because my arm wouldn't work

'I'd work out wearing a brightly coloured headscarf to hide my massive bald patch and scar'

properly. I moved back home so my parents could care for me, but this meant giving up a lot of independence. Exercise allowed me to feel that I was at least helping myself.

First steps

I started with really gentle walking and cycling once a week at my local gym – I had to avoid impact exercise so my brain wouldn't pulsate too much. I'd work out wearing a brightly coloured headscarf because I had a massive bald patch, a huge scar and a bulging shape to my head that wasn't very attractive! Even though it was strange to find the exercise so tiring, I stuck at it and was so proud when after a while I was upgraded to going to the gym twice a week.

I was beginning to regain some of my old strength when my friend Bally told me about told me about a 5K (3 mile) race in London's Hyde Park. I became determined to walk the race with her because I needed a goal and wanted to prove that I was getting fitter and healthier again.

The race and the walking I was doing to prepare for it became my main aim in life, and the day more than lived up to my expectations. The thousands of people taking part and the amount of support we got from the crowds were just amazing. There was a tangible adrenaline buzz in the air and the race seemed to mean so much to everyone there.

Bally and I speed-walked round the course chatting the whole way, and even finished in front of some of the runners, watched proudly by my mum, dad and Bally's boyfriend. I was thrilled to collect my medal and, as I handed over the £1,000 cheque I'd raised for charity to my consultant, he was amazed at how well I'd done. That race gave me support, motivation and self-belief. I was even able to start working again as a film researcher because I'd regained so much confidence. It very quickly became my goal to work up to running the race the following year, and I felt full of hope that I'd be able to keep on improving.

Learning to run again

Two years on from my accident, I had to have another big operation to replace the missing piece of my skull, and had to take barbiturates to prevent me from having fits, which left me feeling pretty lethargic and awful. A few months later, I was given the all-clear to go running for the first time since I'd had my accident, and I decided I'd start training so I could do the 5K (3 mile) race again. The first outing was pretty nerve-wracking. I set off very gently on my own, following a walk/run programme and thinking, 'I hope nothing goes ker-plunk in my head and that bits of my brain don't explode!' I was worried about whether my feet were hitting the ground too hard and sending shockwaves to my brain.

I got a real confidence boost from finding I was fitter than I'd expected, and the longer I was able to run for, the more capable I started to feel. At times I'd be running along wanting to shout out to people, 'Look at me, I can do it, I'm really running!' And although it was hard to motivate myself sometimes as the barbiturates I was taking made me feel apathetic, once I got myself outside, running really helped counteract their effect.

Running with a secret
I completed my second Flora Light Challenge For Women with Bally and my sister in about 30 minutes, and felt incredibly proud of my time. Once again, it was an amazing experience, this time because my sister did it with me, and I realized how much my fitness and health had improved since the previous year. I also loved the fact that anyone watching us run wouldn't have known what had happened to me. I think of my accident as my little secret, unless I choose to tell people about it.

Yearly milestone
The following year I took part again (although I had to walk as I'd injured a ligament) and I'm planning to keep on running the race every year. It's become a milestone on the road to recovery for me, and I even think of it as my own race because it means so much to me. I'm keen to keep getting faster, too!

When I look round and realize lots of people are afraid to try running, I'm so grateful that I dared to give it another go. Taking part in the race has shown me that I can achieve anything I want to if I set my mind to it.

HOW EMMA DID IT
Motivation tip: 'On days when I struggled to motivate myself, I would just try to remember how much running helped me escape from my stresses and frustrations and how much better I felt after I'd run.'
Training tip: 'I followed a walk/run programme, which was a great way back into running. It's really important to take things slowly at first.'

'I WANTED TO RUN SO BADLY, I RAN ON CRUTCHES'

Having only one leg wasn't going to stop NKELE MOSIANE, 38 (centre), from fulfilling her childhood dream of running. That's why this South African from Johannesburg joined a running club and ran three marathons – on crutches.

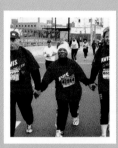

I come from South Africa and in my culture it's traditional to name your child after something you've seen or experienced when giving birth. My name, Nkele, means 'tears' and I've often wondered why my mother called me this. Were they tears of joy at the birth of her first daughter or tears of sorrow because I was born disabled? I don't know why, but I never plucked up the courage to ask her – I like to think it was the former.

I was born with a twisted left foot that had two extra toes and I didn't have a tibia in my left leg so, when I was five, my leg was amputated at the knee. At the age of six, I was fitted with a very crude wood, steel and rubber artificial limb, which enabled me to walk with the aid of crutches.

I hated using crutches so I was really pleased when I got my first proper artificial leg at the age of nine, which meant I could walk unsupported. I found it really difficult being disabled as the other children at my school called me names like 'cripple'. Back then, I would never have dreamed that one day I'd have run five marathons and have a big collection of more than thirty running medals hanging up proudly in my hallway!

Raring to go

One April, when I was working at the Self Help Centre For Paraplegics in Soweto, near Johannesburg, the Achilles Track Club (an organization that aims to encourage disabled people to participate in long-distance running) called and told me it was recruiting members for the new running club it was starting. When I was a schoolgirl, I used to love watching my friends do athletics and yearned to be able to join them. I really hated having to sit on the sidelines watching them run. So when I got the call, I thought to myself, 'At last, this is my chance, I'll give it a try,' and went along to a local sports field with two other women who'd also had their legs amputated, to see if I'd be able to do it. I'd never run so much as a step before so I found running very difficult. My artificial leg was so heavy that I was forced to use crutches, and at first I could only walk.

At every training session I was always the last person to finish, but I persevered because I just loved doing it so much. We started out doing 2K (just over a mile) and it took me 90 minutes to finish. Eventually, I decided to remove my artificial leg as it was holding me back, and just use crutches. Running with crutches was tough as I got really painful blisters on my hands. I developed a style of running that I call the double hop – I'd place both crutches a little way ahead

'I'm not physically challenged …
I see myself as physically challenging as I'm
constantly challenging myself'

of me and then swing my right foot and left stump through. It was a strange way to run!

Crowd support

As an incentive, we entered a 32K (20 mile) race in February the following year. I thoroughly enjoyed it because of all the support I got from the runners and spectators. Their words of encouragement helped me get where I wanted to be – the finish. I got cramp in my foot and thigh and blisters on my hands and foot during the race, but I was elated when I'd done it. I kept looking at my medal and thinking, 'Most able-bodied people don't have a medal, but now I do!'

Spills and thrills

Soon after that first race, I was incredibly excited to be asked whether I'd like to be sponsored by the New York Achilles Track Club to run the New York City Marathon. I had high hopes but that marathon was a real struggle. I was just so nervous, and it was raining and freezing cold. I fell over twice because my crutches slipped on the

wet road, but I gritted my teeth and kept going. I told myself there was no way I could fly all the way from South Africa to America and not finish.

I ran for 750m (½ mile), then walked for 750m, until the final 8K (5 miles), when I ran all the way. I was accompanied by two fantastic American guides who made sure I had everything I needed (they even gave me a roadside massage when I got cramp!). Listening to them and telling them what it's like to live in South Africa helped distract me from the blisters on my hands. The crowd were also amazing – they kept shouting, 'Go! Go! You're almost there!' I loved that crowd because they encouraged me so much. It took me 12 hours and 12 minutes to finish that day, and I felt exhausted but also very proud of what I'd achieved.

Big surprise!

I ended up running the New York City Marathon five times in total, and after I'd completed the third one, I was given a big surprise. I'd been promised a new, lightweight artificial leg before by the New York Achilles Track Club, but each time I'd been bumped on to the waiting list as there'd been other runners whose need was greater than mine. But this time, I was finally given one that was light enough to run with. I was overjoyed as it was really expensive and there was no way I could have afforded to buy such a sophisticated leg myself. At last, I could ditch the crutches and run almost normally – even though I had a slight limp, I felt an incredible sense of freedom. I had to get used to the new leg, which was very painful to use in the beginning. On the places where my stump put pressure on it, I got terrible blisters, but I didn't let that put me off.

I've since run two other New York City Marathons with my new leg, and I've got faster each time. My current personal best time is 8:45 and my next goal is to run it in under eight hours. Along the way, I've also run more than thirty races.

Proud moments

Running has made me what I am – before I used to obsess about my problems but now I just focus on how I'm going to run my next race. It's given me self-belief and confidence: I no longer see myself as physically challenged, but instead see myself as physically challenging as I'm constantly challenging myself. I love encouraging others to run, too. When my friends say they also want to take up running, I say, 'Come along and we'll see what you can do.' I've now helped train the two women who did the New York City Marathon with me – when we all finished, I felt I'd done a really good job. What I'm most proud of, however, is the way I've inspired my daughter. She wasn't a runner, but after she had seen me enter a few races it prompted her to join a running club. Her name is Mapule, which means 'rain', because it was raining when she was born. It's amusing to think that the only thing I don't like about running is doing it when it's raining!

HOW NKELE DID IT

Motivation tip: 'If you're tempted to skip a training session, ask yourself, 'What will I be doing instead?' You'll soon realize that unless you've got really good alternative plans, you'll feel guilty about not going and a lot better if you do.'

Eating tip: 'To give you energy during a run, eat small amounts of foods like sweets, chocolate and bananas.'

'RUNNING HAS BEEN A WONDERFUL REVELATION'

MELANIE WHITTAKER, 40, from Wiltshire, hated running as a child, but it has proved to be an essential part of her recovery from a life-threatening illness.

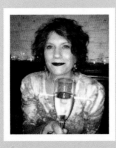

After graduating with a degree in Sociology, my career mainly involved field sales roles and I suppose people would have described me as outgoing and gregarious, with the 'gift of the gab,' as my Mam would say. Then I started a job as a corporate account manager for a telecommunications company. The role came with a lot of responsibility and pressure, and before my illness I could generally be found in a 'whirling dervish' type state. My spare time usually involved socializing, going to the gym and a few glasses of wine!

I had planned to take my fiancé for a long weekend to Amsterdam to celebrate his 40th birthday. Two days before we were due to fly, I was in the office preparing for an important meeting. During the day I was aware of feeling a 'tension headache,' which I put down to the amount of plate spinning I was doing at the time. At around 5pm I excused myself, explaining that I didn't feel tip-top, and planning to finish off at home. By the time I got back it was just after 7pm and I told my fiancé that I needed a half-hour 'nana nap' before finishing my presentation and doing some packing. At this point I was feeling lethargic and my head was pretty fuzzy.

A bolt from the blue

After about 10 minutes I experienced what I can only describe as the feeling of being struck on the head with a cricket bat! Luckily, I screamed (which alerted my fiancé) and then I started sweating and vomiting. My fiancé came upstairs and said my face was contorted and had 'dropped' (he didn't tell me this until a long time later). He rang an ambulance straight away. Thankfully, and to my eternal gratitude, the ambulance crew took me promptly to Macclesfield Hospital where they quickly identified a bleed on the brain.

I had suffered a sub arachnoid brain haemorrhage, which is a type of stroke caused by bleeding in and around the brain. I was then transferred to Salford Royal Hospital, where I underwent eight hours of brain surgery to clip the aneurysm that had burst. Due to the size and location of the bleed the surgical team had to perform a craniotomy and clipping, where a hole is made in the skull and a clip is placed on the base of the aneurysm to stop the blood flow from entering, instead of a coil (which can be inserted via the arteries up into the brain and is the preferred way of dealing with this kind of haemorrhage, as it is less invasive).

A difficult time

My memories of hospital are still really quite bizarre and confused in places.

'When I first got out of hospital everything seemed amplified and quite overwelming'

However, I remember being transferred to a 'normal' ward out of the Neuro Intensive Care unit, and being able to go to the toilet for the first time instead of having a catheter, where I promptly fainted in the cubicle. My friend was visiting me a few days later and as we were speaking I noticed my words were getting all mixed up and what I thought I was saying was not what I could hear coming out of my mouth. It turned out I had suffered a number of mini strokes or vasospasms, so it was back up to ICU for me, for a spinal fluid drain and a shot of drugs directly into my brain to minimize damage. In total I was hospital for nearly two months.

System overload
When I first got out of hospital, everything seemed amplified and quite overwhelming. In addition I was absolutely shattered. For the first 12 months of recovery, I really struggled with the 'normal' things in life. Of course initially I was tired and slept a lot of the time. Eventually I came to identify some of the fatigue as being 'brain tired': you can really feel your brain working and how hard it has to do so, and frankly it is exhausting! It quickly became

apparent that my short-term memory was not what it was and also I really struggled with things like having the TV on if my husband was talking to me at the same time, or being in a supermarket, where all I seemed to hear was the bleeping of tills, hustle and bustle of people and a cacophony of things 'coming at me' all at once.

Going to the gym was pretty impossible too, as it is a place where large numbers of people are all doing different activities, music is playing and people are talking. Eventually, I was told that my memory, concentration and divided attention had been affected by the haemorrhage, a common feature of brain injury.

Coping with life
Although I am extremely blessed and lucky – I'm alive after all – and apart from the dent in my head, you cannot see any visible signs of the damage that had been done to my brain. However, I still have a number of issues that massively affect 'real life' now, and along with various other areas of support, it was advised I take exercise to help me cope.

I was 37 when the haemorrhage occurred, and I am now 40, and I can say with conviction that I disliked running with a passion. The memory of cross country runs at school and sprinting on sports day filled me with horror. My specialist neuropsychologist was keen to get me participating in group situations, and more importantly getting my heart going and I was struggling to find something, apart from walking, that I could do.

A friend recommended we go for a run one day and we ran for about 1.6K (1 mile) along one of the local trails by the river. As it turned out I quite enjoyed it: there was no noise, no pressure, just lovely countryside and peace. The next week my friend suggested the beginner's group she ran with. This terrified me but the group leader called me up that day and we had a really good chat about what the group did, and my challenges. His simple question 'What have you got to lose, except an hour of your time?', struck a chord. So I went that Saturday and have never looked back.

Finding some peace

Joining the group allowed me to be outside, interacting with others, but at the same time managing my issues and achieving amazing 'head space'. We are incredibly lucky in Macclesfield to be able to run completely off road (as I am unable to deal with cars or traffic without becoming overwhelmed or 'brain tired'). Being in the gorgeous countryside, breathing and running, is truly liberating, calming and peace inducing. From my starting point in September 2012, when I could barely run 1K (2/3 mile), I now regularly run 3 times a week between 6 and 10K (3.7–6 miles). It's incredible, and I miss it like mad if I can't get out.

Living day to day is still a huge challenge for me and I began a return to work, very part time and slowly, last year. In time, and if I can find a suitable one, I would love to run some timed events to raise money for the brain and spine injury charity that helped me initially. My group leader Neil and his wife Alison, and their ultra supportive group have been amazing and I can't thank them enough.

HOW MELANIE DID IT

Motivation tip: 'Get a running "buddy" or buddies: although I like running alone, having someone with you is safer and means you are more likely to carry on and run further yourself!'

Eating tip: 'I like running in the morning and always have a banana an hour before I run and porridge afterwards.'

'I DO THINGS SIGHTED RUNNERS CAN'T'

JOHNNIE DEMAS, 56, from Johannesburg, South Africa, lost his sight in a vicious gang attack more than 30 years ago. Yet 11 years later, he took his first tentative steps as a blind runner, holding one end of a handkerchief while a sighted runner held the other …

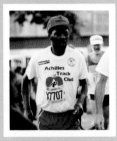

I've been blind for more than 30 years. I live in Johannesburg, which can be a very violent city, and my life changed for ever one day in November 1974, when, aged 26, I was attacked by a gang, who mistook me for someone else. I suffered multiple stab wounds and my skull was fractured by a brick. After the attack, I had brain surgery and was unconscious for 45 days. The doctors didn't think I'd survive and feared I'd be brain damaged. Waking up from that coma was terrible – when I found that all I could see was blackness, I knew I'd gone blind, and that I'd be blind for life. I felt rage at the gang for doing such a thing to me and I also felt helpless as there was nothing I could do about it.

Big adjustment

It truly was the hardest time in my life. I felt so miserable and found adjusting to being blind very difficult. I felt I had no future because, as a bricklayer, there was no way I could continue with my job. I was single at the time but I thank God for my family, who helped me through.

Life-changing moment

For six years I was unable to work and I lived off a disability pension, but then I managed to get a job glueing handles into paper carrier bags at the Services for the Blind and Visually Handicapped organization. It didn't pay very much but I enjoyed it. I began to feel less depressed because I met other people who'd also once been able to see but were now blind. Before that I'd thought I was the only person in the world that this had happened to.

My life changed again one day when Denis Tabakin, who works for the Achilles Track Club (an organization that aims to encourage disabled people to participate in long-distance running), came to my workplace and gave a talk about running. He said it was possible for blind people to run by holding on to one end of a handkerchief while a sighted person held the other. Quite a few of us were tempted to give running a go, and so, accompanied by Denis and two social workers, we went off to try it out.

In the beginning I found running really scary as I was terrified of smacking into a lamp-post or tree. It was hard learning to put my total trust in my guide. Eventually, however, I got used to it – I learnt not to worry about where I was putting my feet and just run in faith. I found my hearing became more acute as I had to listen out for traffic and other runners, and I also began to 'read' the road with my feet.

'When I woke up from the coma, all I could see was blackness and I knew I'd be blind for life'

Over several weeks we built up to doing 5K (3 miles) and then we entered an 8K (5 mile) fun run. It was my first race and I really enjoyed it. When I won a bottle of Scotch whisky in the prize draw, I thought, 'I'll definitely be back for more!'

Racing ahead

Our group of eight runners eventually joined the Rocky Road Runners Club, which had lots of members willing to be guides, and I'm a member to this day. I gradually increased the distances I was running and then began to wonder whether I'd be able to do the Johannesburg Marathon. I trained really hard and did it in 4:24.

After that, I began to think of myself as a real runner and became totally hooked on running! Instead of spending my weekends moping around the house feeling sorry for myself, I entered races most Sundays, met lots of new people and made new friends.

Soon, I realized marathons weren't enough and I set my sights on the Comrades ultra-marathon, an 89K (55.6 mile) race. With my guide, Richard Shakenovsky, I managed to do it in 10:29. It never crossed my mind that we wouldn't finish and I was positive the whole time. You have to be mentally strong to tackle a distance as long as Comrades. Finishing felt so great – I simply couldn't quite believe I'd run 89K. I've run it every year since and love doing it.

That year was also memorable in another way because I married my wife, Ida, whom I'd met at work. She's blind, too, and even though she's not a runner herself, she's really proud of what I've achieved. We have two children, Lorimee and Richard, who's named after my first guide. I manage to combine running with family life by running 9K (5.6 miles) before work three times a week. I meet my running partner, Gerald Fox, at 5.45am and we run from there to work. On Sundays I go for a longer run.

Great guides

I've had several guides (we call them pilots!) over the years and they've all become close friends. We take turns setting the pace, which can be frustrating at times, and if one of us needs the loo, the other simply has to wait for him. I'm not a talkative person but I like running with a guide, especially a chatty one, because it helps keep my mind off how far we have to go. My guide tells me how the other runners are doing and describes the scenery so I can imagine what it looks like and appreciate it, too. He also warns me of any obstacles and tells me if there's a hill ahead. But if he loses concentration, it can have disastrous consequences. One year, when I was running the Two Oceans Marathon in Cape Town, my guide started chatting to some other runners just as we passed a water table. I slipped on the discarded cups and injured my knees really badly. It didn't stop me finishing, but he felt terribly guilty afterwards.

Marathon man

Why do I love running? Well, it makes me feel good and has helped me have a better self-image. I used to be overweight but I've lost 8kg (1st 4lb) and look great. I'm also proud of all my achievements and think it's wonderful that I can do something that many sighted runners haven't done. One such achievement was doing the Golden Reef 100 Miler (160K), which I ran to raise funds for a charity that cares for abused and HIV-positive children. I ran most of the way but

walked up the hills and it took me 22 hours and 58 minutes! So far, I've done 40 marathons and 16 consecutive Comrades, a record for a blind runner, and my goal is to run 20. When other runners call me 'The Marathon Man' or say, 'Here's the Comrades King!,' it feels fantastic.'

Whole new world

Running has totally transformed my life. I've made life-long friends with my guides and it even helped me get the job I have now.

I wonder if I'd be a runner today if I hadn't been blinded. Running has opened up a whole new world for me. It's helped me feel that I'm just as good as anyone else – it's just that I can't see. I love it when fellow runners say to me, "You're an amazing man – you've got all the excuses in the world not to run but you still do it."

HOW JOHNNIE DID IT

Motivation tip: 'Try to do your run first thing to make sure you don't get distracted by other commitments during the day.'

Training tip: 'Run with a friend because you can't let them down. I meet my partner at a certain place each time and I know I can't let him stand there and not turn up!'

KICK OFF YOUR TRAINERS, PUT YOUR
FEET UP AND POUR YOURSELF A
DRINK – IT'S TIME TO CELEBRATE
JUST HOW FAR YOU'VE COME ...

11. GET CELEBRATING

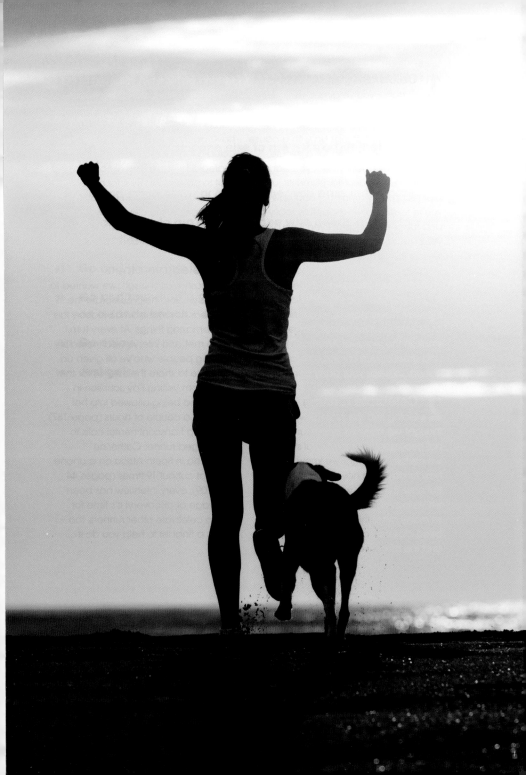

WE'VE DONE OUR BIT AND NOW IT'S
YOUR TURN TO GET WRITING. USE THE
ULTIMATE 6-MONTH RUNNING DIARY
TO DIARIZE AND ANALYZE EVERY RUN.
GOOD LUCK — AND KEEP ON RUNNING!

12. GET
SCRIBBLING

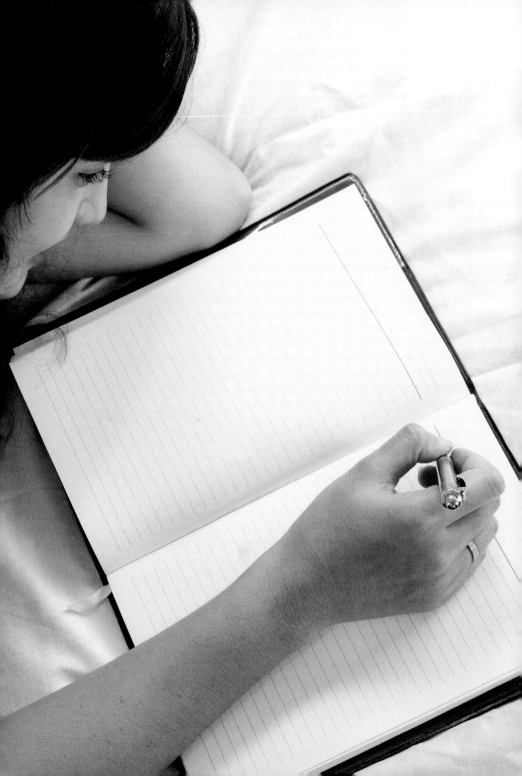

YOUR ULTIMATE 6-MONTH RUNNING DIARY

Nothing's more satisfying than looking back on your training to see how far you've come.

Each day you'll be making small, almost invisible improvements, until one day you'll wake up and realize that goals you once thought were impossible (running three times a week, running 5K/3 miles in under 30 minutes or even running a marathon) are either within reach or already ticked off on your 'Been there, done that' list.

Each time you go for a run, fill in the running diary on the pages that follow – and then review your progress regularly to see whether you can spot anything that will help you get even better, and adjust your training accordingly. So, for example, if you always have Euphoric runs on grass but Hellish ones on the treadmill, schedule more runs in the sun. (If you've forgotten exactly what those little Mood-O-Meter symbols mean, turn back to page 72 for the lowdown.)

Here's how to fill in the running diary – use whichever categories are useful to you, and feel free to ignore the rest!

- **Date** Write down the date of when you did your session.

- **Time** Write down how long you went out running for.

- **Distance** (optional) If you know it, write down how far you ran in kilometres or miles.

- **Type of run** Did you do an ordinary run or did you do some speed-training (such as intervals)?

- **Where I ran** Write down whether you ran on a track, road, grass, pavement, trail or treadmill (if you ran on a treadmill, make a note of the incline and speed you ran at).

- **Mood before/during/after** Simply draw the facial expression that best applies to you on the icons provided. Use the key at the top of the page to remind you of the options.

Hellish   **Indifferent**   **Up and down**   **Good**   **Euphoric**

Date	Time	Distance	Type of run	Where I ran	Mood before	Mood during	Mood after
Mon							
Tues							
Weds							
Thurs							
Fri							
Sat							
Sun							

Date	Time	Distance	Type of run	Where I ran	Mood before	Mood during	Mood after
Mon							
Tues							
Weds							
Thurs							
Fri							
Sat							
Sun							

'It's not about being first or last, it's about having the courage to finish the race'

Catherine Mokwena, administrator

Hellish　 **Indifferent**　 **Up and down**　 **Good**　 **Euphoric**

Date	Time	Distance	Type of run	Where I ran	Mood before	Mood during	Mood after
Mon							
Tues							
Weds							
Thurs							
Fri							
Sat							
Sun							

Date	Time	Distance	Type of run	Where I ran	Mood before	Mood during	Mood after
Mon							
Tues							
Weds							
Thurs							
Fri							
Sat							
Sun							

'Be your own hero, it's cheaper than a movie ticket'

Doug Horton, science-fiction author

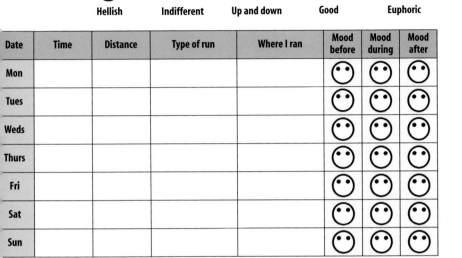

Date	Time	Distance	Type of run	Where I ran	Mood before	Mood during	Mood after
Mon							
Tues							
Weds							
Thurs							
Fri							
Sat							
Sun							

Date	Time	Distance	Type of run	Where I ran	Mood before	Mood during	Mood after
Mon							
Tues							
Weds							
Thurs							
Fri							
Sat							
Sun							

'All things excellent are as difficult as they are rare'

Benedict de Spinoza, philosopher

Hellish   **Indifferent**   **Up and down**   **Good**   **Euphoric**

Date	Time	Distance	Type of run	Where I ran	Mood before	Mood during	Mood after
Mon							
Tues							
Weds							
Thurs							
Fri							
Sat							
Sun							

Date	Time	Distance	Type of run	Where I ran	Mood before	Mood during	Mood after
Mon							
Tues							
Weds							
Thurs							
Fri							
Sat							
Sun							

'The best preparation for tomorrow is doing your best today'

Henry Jackson Brown Jr, writer

Hellish   **Indifferent**   **Up and down**   **Good**   **Euphoric**

Date	Time	Distance	Type of run	Where I ran	Mood before	Mood during	Mood after
Mon					☺	☺	☺
Tues					☺	☺	☺
Weds					☺	☺	☺
Thurs					☺	☺	☺
Fri					☺	☺	☺
Sat					☺	☺	☺
Sun					☺	☺	☺

Date	Time	Distance	Type of run	Where I ran	Mood before	Mood during	Mood after
Mon					☺	☺	☺
Tues					☺	☺	☺
Weds					☺	☺	☺
Thurs					☺	☺	☺
Fri					☺	☺	☺
Sat					☺	☺	☺
Sun					☺	☺	☺

> ### 'We can't all be heroes, because somebody has to sit on the curb and clap as they go by'
> **Will Rogers,** writer

Hellish	Indifferent	Up and down	Good	Euphoric

Date	Time	Distance	Type of run	Where I ran	Mood before	Mood during	Mood after
Mon							
Tues							
Weds							
Thurs							
Fri							
Sat							
Sun							

Date	Time	Distance	Type of run	Where I ran	Mood before	Mood during	Mood after
Mon							
Tues							
Weds							
Thurs							
Fri							
Sat							
Sun							

'Everyone runs the same distance in a race – if you look at the runners at the back, they're trying just as hard as those at the front – it's just that some people can go faster than others'

Pippa Major, e-commerce development manager

Hellish **Indifferent** **Up and down** **Good** **Euphoric**

Date	Time	Distance	Type of run	Where I ran	Mood before	Mood during	Mood after
Mon					☺	☺	☺
Tues					☺	☺	☺
Weds					☺	☺	☺
Thurs					☺	☺	☺
Fri					☺	☺	☺
Sat					☺	☺	☺
Sun					☺	☺	☺

Date	Time	Distance	Type of run	Where I ran	Mood before	Mood during	Mood after
Mon					☺	☺	☺
Tues					☺	☺	☺
Weds					☺	☺	☺
Thurs					☺	☺	☺
Fri					☺	☺	☺
Sat					☺	☺	☺
Sun					☺	☺	☺

'The only place where success comes before work is in the dictionary'

Vidal Sassoon, legendary hairdresser

Hellish   **Indifferent**   **Up and down**   **Good**   **Euphoric**

Date	Time	Distance	Type of run	Where I ran	Mood before	Mood during	Mood after
Mon					😐	😐	😐
Tues					😐	😐	😐
Weds					😐	😐	😐
Thurs					😐	😐	😐
Fri					😐	😐	😐
Sat					😐	😐	😐
Sun					😐	😐	😐

Date	Time	Distance	Type of run	Where I ran	Mood before	Mood during	Mood after
Mon					😐	😐	😐
Tues					😐	😐	😐
Weds					😐	😐	😐
Thurs					😐	😐	😐
Fri					😐	😐	😐
Sat					😐	😐	😐
Sun					😐	😐	😐

'Running is like medicine – sometimes it tastes good, sometimes it doesn't, but it always makes you feel better afterwards'

Gail Marcus, managing director

Hellish   **Indifferent**   **Up and down**   **Good**   **Euphoric**

Date	Time	Distance	Type of run	Where I ran	Mood before	Mood during	Mood after
Mon					😐	😐	😐
Tues					😐	😐	😐
Weds					😐	😐	😐
Thurs					😐	😐	😐
Fri					😐	😐	😐
Sat					😐	😐	😐
Sun					😐	😐	😐

Date	Time	Distance	Type of run	Where I ran	Mood before	Mood during	Mood after
Mon					😐	😐	😐
Tues					😐	😐	😐
Weds					😐	😐	😐
Thurs					😐	😐	😐
Fri					😐	😐	😐
Sat					😐	😐	😐
Sun					😐	😐	😐

'Remember, you can run and many cannot and will not run.
Some people have never known what it's like to run.
Make the most of it while you can'

Frank Horwill, international running coach

Hellish   **Indifferent**   **Up and down**   **Good**   **Euphoric**

Date	Time	Distance	Type of run	Where I ran	Mood before	Mood during	Mood after
Mon							
Tues							
Weds							
Thurs							
Fri							
Sat							
Sun							

Date	Time	Distance	Type of run	Where I ran	Mood before	Mood during	Mood after
Mon							
Tues							
Weds							
Thurs							
Fri							
Sat							
Sun							

'It's hard to beat a person who never gives up'

Babe Ruth, baseball legend

Hellish   **Indifferent**   **Up and down**   **Good**   **Euphoric**

Date	Time	Distance	Type of run	Where I ran	Mood before	Mood during	Mood after
Mon							
Tues							
Weds							
Thurs							
Fri							
Sat							
Sun							

Date	Time	Distance	Type of run	Where I ran	Mood before	Mood during	Mood after
Mon							
Tues							
Weds							
Thurs							
Fri							
Sat							
Sun							

'The vision of a champion is someone who is bent over, drenched in sweat, at the point of exhaustion, when no one else is watching'

Anson Dorrance, women's football coach

Hellish   **Indifferent**   **Up and down**   **Good**   **Euphoric**

Date	Time	Distance	Type of run	Where I ran	Mood before	Mood during	Mood after
Mon							
Tues							
Weds							
Thurs							
Fri							
Sat							
Sun							

Date	Time	Distance	Type of run	Where I ran	Mood before	Mood during	Mood after
Mon							
Tues							
Weds							
Thurs							
Fri							
Sat							
Sun							

'Most look up and admire the stars.
A champion climbs a mountain and grabs one'
Henry Jackson Brown Jr, writer

MY PERSONAL BEST LIST

▶▶

Knowing you're getting faster can be an incredible motivator. Record your personal best times (PBs) here to see how much you've improved.

Best time for 1.6km/1 mile

Time and date _____

Time and date _____

Time and date _____

Time and date _____

Time and date _____

Time and date _____

Best time for 10K/6 miles

Time and date _____

Time and date _____

Time and date _____

Time and date _____

Time and date _____

Time and date _____

Best time for 5K/3 miles

Time and date _____

Time and date _____

Time and date _____

Time and date _____

Time and date _____

Time and date _____

Best time for a half-marathon (21km/13.1 miles)

Time and date _____

Time and date _____

Time and date _____

Time and date _____

Time and date _____

Time and date _____

Best time for 8km/5 miles

Time and date _____

Time and date _____

Time and date _____

Time and date _____

Time and date _____

Time and date _____

Best time for a marathon (42km/26.2 miles)

Time and date _____

Time and date _____

Time and date _____

Time and date _____

Time and date _____

Time and date _____

CONTACT US ...

If this book has inspired you to take up running, or helped you get better at it, we'd really love to hear from you. Email Lisa at quiet.medicine@gmail.com or Susie at susiewhalley@hotmail.com and you may even be featured in a future edition of this book. To book fitness-motivation hypnotherapy sessions with Lisa, visit www.quiet-medicine.co.uk.

READ THESE ...

Adore Yourself Slim by Lisa Jackson, Simon & Schuster, 2011
The Courage To Start by John Bingham, Prentice Hall & IBD, 2003
The Run-Walk-Run Method by Jeff Galloway, Meyer & Meyer Sport, 2013
Lore of Running by Tim Noakes, Human Kinetics, 2002
The Complete Guide To Sports Nutrition by Anita Bean, Bloomsbury Sport, 2013
Eat Smart, Play Hard by Liz Applegate, Rodale Books, 2001
Marathon Woman by Kathrine Switzer, Da Capo Press, 2009
Born To Run by Christopher McDougall, Profile Books, 2010
My Life On The Run by Bart Yasso, Rodale Press, 2009
26.2 Marathon Stories by Kathrine Switzer and Roger Robinson, Rodale, 2006
Running Crazy by Helen Summer, John Blake Publishing, 2013
Runner's World magazine – to subscribe, visit www.runnersworld.co.uk
Women's Running UK – to subscribe, visit www.womensrunninguk.co.uk
Men's Running UK – to subscribe, visit www.mensrunninguk.co.uk

VISIT THESE ...

www.sportsister.com, a website that features up-to-the-minute news on all women's sports, including running
www.trekandrun.com, a website that features coverage (and amazing video footage) of races around the world

RUN THESE ...

• Parkrun (free, weekly, 5K timed runs around the world): www.parkrun.org.uk
• RunEngland: www.runengland.info
• Race For Life (Cancer Research UK's series of 5K and 10K women-only events raising funds for cancer research): www.raceforlife.org
• To enter most UK races online, visit www.runnersworld.co.uk

A BIG THANK YOU TO ...

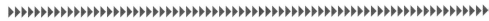

▶▶ Katie Hewett, Laura Russell, Lisa Tai, Jenny Wheatley, Krissy Mallett, Miriam Hyslop, Helen Ponting, Abby Franklin, and all at Anova Books, past and present, as well our wonderful colleagues at Hearst Magazines (in particular Rachel Boston, Kelly Flood, Marianne de Vries and Kelly Moseley) who worked on the first two editions of *Running Made Easy* and were so supportive and crucial in getting the book up and running.

▶▶ Thanks to the experts who shared their expertise with us. Special thanks to Suzy Fitt (www.fittlife.com), Dr Dorian Dugmore, Georgie Gladwyn at PhysioCentral, London, Jon Roberts, Jane Wake, Sammy Margo, the experts who designed our running plans (Kirsty O'Neill, Joe Dunbar, Andy Ellis and Prof Tim Noakes), and to Prof Andrew Prentice for information about body-fat composition.

▶▶ Thanks, too, to all our wonderful case studies and the organizations that put us in touch with them: the London Marathon (www.london-marathon.co.uk), Cancer Research UK (www.cancerresearchuk.org), Shelter (www.shelter.org.uk), Mind (www.mind.org.uk), Denis Tabakin at the Achilles Track Club (www.achillesinternational.org), Slimming World (www.slimmingworld.com), Weight Watchers (www.weightwatchers.co.uk), Vittel, the American Cancer Society (www.cancer.org), Action On Addiction (www.aona.co.uk) and Victoria Wallis (www.thamesfitness.co.uk), RunEngland and Running 4 Women.

▶▶ And lastly, thanks to the hundreds of really enthusiastic runners from around the world who sent in written contributions and to the many people who bought the first two editions of this book, used The 60-Second-Secret Plan to become runners and loved it so much that they turned many of their friends and family into runners, too!

Lisa and Susie

INDEX